Fighting for My Future

A personal battle against terminal cancer

David Cosgrave

First published in the United Kingdom in 2019

ISBN: 978-1-9160030-0-2 (Print)
ISBN: 978-1-9160030-1-9 (Kindle)
ISBN: 978-1-9160030-2-6 (ePub)

Typeset by Ian Hughes, www.mousematdesign.com

Printed and bound by Createspace

Dedication

This book is dedicated to my wonderful son, Garreth.
He has been with me on every step of my journey,
as I battle with this horrible cancer,
through the good times and the bad times.

Acknowledgements

I am deeply indebted to the following people for all their help:
Theresa Guerrero-Urbano (my Consultant); Hannah; Claire; Laura (CNS); Cate; Gemma; everyone in Guys Oncology; Judith and everyone in Chemotherapy Co-ordination; all nurses in Guys Chemotherapy Department; all staff in Guys Radiotherapy Department; Guys patient transport; St Thomas' CT and Pet Scan Department; Guys Pain team; Doctors and nurses in the PRUH (Princess Royal University Hospital; Stacey and Lynne in PRUH Radiology; PRUH Surgeons; all in Medical 9, especially Maria from Corinth (Greece); Medical 6, especially Eva and Jackie; Yvonne, my Dietician at the Harris Hospice clinic; Starr my gastric band surgical assist; Nina my Savoy Ventures driver, Fola and Michelle in The New Cancer Centre patient transport; my son Garreth; my family in Ireland (my sister Mary and her family for the non-stop, without-fail, daily phone calls that kept me going; my brother Liam and his family; my sister-in-law Catherine; my family in the UK and in particular my cousin Mary Mullally for the caring contact etc; Dr Chris M (my previous GP); staff in The Family Surgery at Green St Green; the great residents where I live in Bassetts Way BR6; for my great neighbours Ian and Anne; the Kennedy family; Ariane; Bruce and their family; Vanessa; Mark and their family; Jane G; Roman and Tanya; Lorraine and Paul S; John and Cheryl; Julie B; my good friend and neighbour Paul Sealey; my neighbour Becs; my good friend Anne Cerase from St. Swithun's RC Church; Adrian and his family of BVTC; all in St Christopher's; my good friend Diane Abbott in Liverpool, for the all-important phone contact; Chrys and Maria Kokkinos for over 20 years of friendship; my friend of many years Ernest Venes, in Lyttelton, New Zealand; the Kantarakias family in Skiathos Greece; Shan in Perth, Western Australia, who has been my great friend of many years; Barbara and Sandra in Boston; Willie and Carole, Phil and Jackie O'Reilly and their family; my bus 'family' in New Cross Bus Garage; my mum and dad for raising me and for teaching me, all those years ago, the rightful values of life and caring for my fellow human beings.

If I have forgotten anybody, then I truly apologise.

Foreword

Hi all, I feel that it is only right that I should explain my reasons for writing this book. I worked for over 20 years as a bus driver and I loved it. My life came crashing down though,in late 2013, when I was diagnosed with cancer. It soon became clear that I was going to die from it, and the prognosis was 12 to 18 months to live. Nobody ever expects it to happen to them but that day was my turn. The treatments of Chemo and Radiotherapy began very quickly. I had always kept an exact diary of my work on the buses, so I decided to change it to a daily record of my cancer journey instead. From that diary I had the idea to publish it as a book. This journal tells everything, exactly as it happened to me. Some of the details are quite gory, some are sad, others are humourous. All have been included in the book, with nothing omitted. I wrote the book so that any fellow cancer sufferers can read it and be aware of what could happen to them along the way, if they undertake a similar journey to mine. I also wrote it as if I am speaking and please take note that the occasional spelling or grammar mistakes may have crept in along the way. Please forgive these. I hope you read it to the end and understand my reason for undertaking it. I am so glad that I have written it and also been able finish it. It is my first attempt at writing anything like this. Finally, by all means contact me if you are concerned about anything concerning cancer or its associated problems. You can get in touch via Facebook (David Cosgrave, London Central Bus Company).

God Bless you all, Dave..x

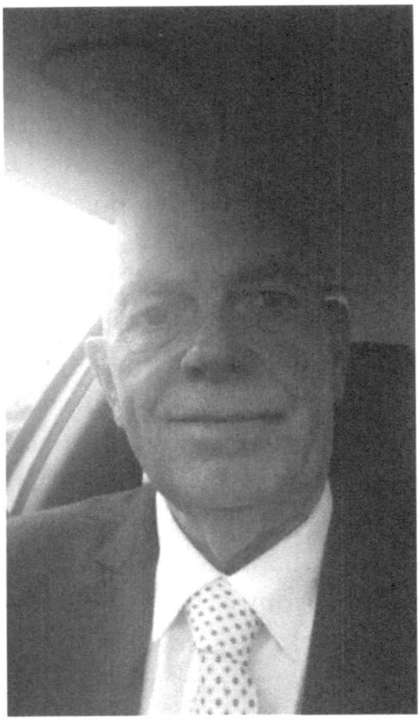 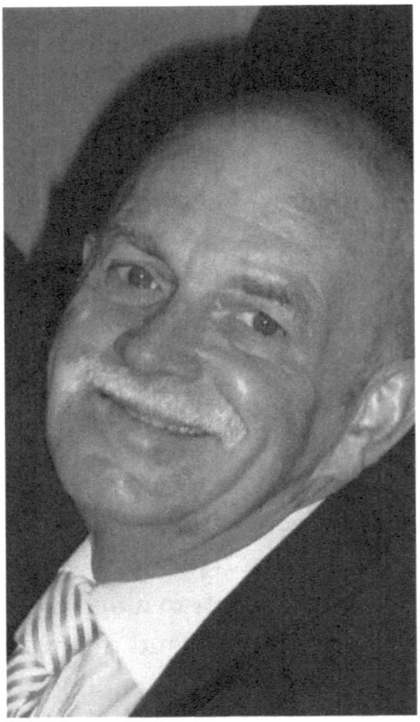

These two photos were taken just before my accidental fall and show how healthy I looked and felt.

Thursday September 5th 2013

On Thursday, September 5th, 2013, I drove to work as usual to New Cross Bus Garage, for 614 duty on Route 436. Sign on time would have been 5.59am but as I was needing a parking space I got there shortly after 5am. I think it was a slightly foggy misty morning but I was looking forward to my day as I loved my job as a bus driver. I joined in June 1994 as a bus conductor and began driving in 1996. Initially, I drove the Routemaster Buses and eventually with other bus types on every route from the garage. The canteen upstairs had a wall on the north side where all senior drivers sat. I remember when I joined first thinking, "Jesus, when will I get to sit on that f*****g side of the canteen" I knew it would come eventually but it would be many years. The more drivers and conductors were discouraged from staying in the job, the bigger my chances increased if they were senior and places were taken on the seats by the wall. I now know that any senior staff that sat there, viewed and discussed the rest of the canteen. I'm sure I was talked about many a time but my day came eventually and I observed and talked about the newbies and how long they would last. We heard them chatting about the crazy things that happened on the road "This guy cut me up, that guy wouldn't pay his fare" Usual stories that we all had but it was old news now and we just got on with it. Every day was different on the buses. Every minute was different. London has many crazy f*****s in it, as well as lovely people. I treated everyone well, nothing bothered me after my 2007 heart attack, it's not worth it. I would have done anything for anyone to make their day or life better.

Anyhow, I parked my car and walked on the pavement which was running alongside a wall at the back of the parked up Bendy Buses. Before I knew it, I had tripped up and fallen to the ground. I must have been knocked out for a minute or so but when I opened my eyes, I realised that I was lying on my right side but actually lying against the wall of the pavement. I was dazed and confused. I was trying to work out what happened and how I ended up where I was. I managed to grab the metal barrier that was the culprit and I found my right leg caught inside a hoop on the pavement that secured the barrier in place. I gradually realised that something bad had happened. I opened my eyes a bit more and then noticed that the lighting was poor and that this poor lighting from the light on a tall pole was partly obscured by vegetation, possibly a tree branch, bushes or something like that. I just knew that it was not as it should be and I was injured and bleeding because of it. I realised that I had tripped on that hoop and hence the injury. I managed to get to my feet and found my work bag. I then also realised that in that part of the garage at night, foxes scavenge for any waste food left lying around in the empty buses or on the ground after being swept from the buses by the cleaners. I was therefore lucky that no wandering foxes had pissed on me. If I had been there for longer, there was an increased chance that it would have happened to me. I felt warm liquid running down my face as I stood up. I put my hand to my head and as I took it away, I looked at it and it was red. It was red with my blood and it was a lot. I knew that I needed help so I decided to get across the garage yard and look for someone to help me. I slowly staggered across the garage yard towards the main entrance. The blood was still flowing freely and had wet my shirt and was now spattering on the ground. I must have looked a right state in my high vis jacket in yellow and a white shirt spattered with blood from a head wound and I was still inside the garage. What a great start to a day. I remember all my work colleagues being concerned for me. It was a manic time of the day with some night drivers finishing and signing off any defects on their buses from the night shift and so, so many day drivers now signing on for their day shifts. I was to have been one of those day drivers but it was highly likely now that I would somehow have to go to a hospital to have my injury treated, maybe even have stitches in my head wound. I was taken behind the counter to a back room and my cut etc was treated and dressed by Nick Burnett who was the trained First Aider there at the time. Little did I know then but finally my days in New Cross Garage were coming to an end with over 20 years service under my belt. Over the next few months my life would undergo a complete change around.

Anyhow, Nick dressed my wound and we waited for the ambulance. I was eventually taken to Kings College Hospital in Denmark Hill and admitted to A and E as a patient with a severe Head injury. I was going to spend the rest of the day or longer in Kings College Hospital. During the day and after the wound had been treated further, X Rays were taken and I was kept under observation all day and evening. I was finally discharged in the late evening and I then made my way down to the bus stop in Camberwell Green. It was there while waiting for any bus that would get me to New Cross Gate and the Bus Garage that I spoke to my Garage Operating Manager on my mobile and was told to "take tomorrow off as a sick day". I was also told me not to worry as it would not affect my Attendance Bonus. I always got on with my OM and their family since the day I joined the Garage back in 1994. This bonus was actually a great incentive that encouraged any staff not to take days off sick etc. I was now feeling tired and anxious to get home. Little did I know that the next few weeks and months would be a living f*****g nightmare. The company ignored my 20 years of loyalty to them as I will explain shortly. I was also about to change to health problems which were going to have a life changing outcome. My own personal living hell was about to be unleashed on me and there was absolutely nothing I could do to control it. Before all this was going to happen, lets go back to my day of injury and recovering on Friday September 6th 2013. The next day was Saturday September 7th, I was not one to milk the situation as I returned to work with a headache and a scar on my head and face. I was doing 614 duty on the 436 route Saturday, times signed on at 7.57am. The day of the accident, I still remember tripping because of the poor lighting and I caught my foot on a ground hoop as part of the barrier. It appears that now the company had already decided to act ahead of any possible queries that I had about the cause of my accident.

On Thursday September 12th my duty was suddenly changed in advance to be a 7am Stand By as I had to see my management in their office. I am a decent human being but for the purposes of this book there was someone in head office and well away from the Bus Garage who I assume made sure that I was facing a disciplinary action because I fell and incase I was going to sue the Company on Health and Safety issues, possibly leading to my fall and injury. I never had any intention of doing that and this is still the case. After 20 years of loyal service someone in head office had decided that I was to be disciplined. It f*****g annoys me that this was happening to me and I do not know who wanted it done. Let me also say that now I don't want to know who they are, but I was disciplined. It was not the fault of the person who disciplined me. I hold no grudge on that person as they were probably told to do it. At the meeting on Thursday, I was disciplined and given a final written warning for the following absurd reason. The pavement where I fell and badly injured myself was, in someone's opinion, not a valid usable pavement until after a certain time. Therefore it was decided that I walked there illegally and I put the company in danger of legal action by having an actual accident. Poor lighting caused me to trip and smash my head yet I was disciplined in case I sued for compensation. What a bad thing to do to me. When I first joined, I was always told that the company always looked on staff as a number and treated people bad. I was disappointed and annoyed when disciplined because I was never going to sue then. They certainly were beginning to live up to the reputation that I was told about. Someone in Head office is a pretender and a fake. I want to say to all my management despite the disciplinary, thank you for all that you done for me while I was employed by the company. This is where that matter ends as regards disciplinary but the injury had consequences. Monday September 23rd 2013. I have a gastric band since 2007 when I was 24 stone in weight. Now I am about 12 stone and 7 lbs. I had my gastric band checked out today in the Princess Royal University Hospital (PRUH) by Starr my gastro team surgical assistant. All is well with that. My work on the buses continues as normal and all is well at work, but during the last few days of September into October I noticed a lump on the outside of the left side of my neck. I had my 56th Birthday as usual on the 7th of October. Work was good and on Friday October 11th at 5.35pm, I had my flu jab. Over the next few days more lumps gradually appeared on the same left side of my neck. On the following Friday I met up with Lizzie for a coffee and a chat. Lizzie is a good friend of mine from the Garage. Anyhow, it was becoming obvious that the lumps on that left side were not going away and actually some new lumps were now starting to appear on the right side of my neck.

My work however, continued as uninterrupted as possible. At this stage there was no reason to do otherwise. I was even putting in requests at work allocation to do overtime and work some rest days. I cannot remember when, but I made an appointment to see my GP Dr Chris about these lumps. At that appointment he explained that he was very concerned. He referred me to Dr T in the Princess Royal University Hospital as the lumps did not appear to be cysts. On November 4th 2013, I attended the PRUH (Princess Royal University Hospital) at 2.50pm for an ENT appointment. It was my day off from work and it was probably at this appointment that my life was in the very early stages of being altered forever when he mentioned that terrifying, scary, nasty, life-changing word called Cancer. I thought "what the hell is going to happen now" In my mind I thought that this could have been delayed if I had worked on my day off but then it would have happened anyway at a later date. Now I had to stop putting things off. I knew then that I would not be leaving the room just with that. There was far more to come from Dr T and after I wanted to know more, he didn't hold back. Dr T then said to me that not only did I have cancer but it was possible that I had cancer of the lymph glands He also requested a biopsy and a scan. I could feel a cry welling up inside me. A scary lip quiver started and there was nothing I could do to stop it happening. Dr T knew what was going on in my mind, as he probably had been in this position with other people numerous times before even though it was completely new to me. While all this was going on in his room, I had to leave the "safety" of his consultation room and go out to the outside world. I was on my own and suddenly the previously safe outside world was a very scary place. I just burst out crying in this now scary and lonely world. I could see people looking at me like I was a mental case. I couldn't ask anybody for help and eventually my slightly loud crying eased off.

I left the hospital and went in the direction of the car park where my car was parked. As soon as I was inside the car, all crazy things went through my mind again. I thought why me, this is wrong and what happens next. I knew I was back in work tomorrow or so and that would take my mind off of it for a while as I waited for dates of Biopsies and scans. I was right, work took my mind off it and of course I told my family, friends and colleagues what happened, what was going to happen next and then of course I was being brave by saying that nobody knows yet until the scans and biopsies are done and results come back. Somehow, I had a slight feeling that Dr T was right and by asking him for the full picture, I was partially prepared. On Sunday November 17th there was an Anniversary mass for my late wife Joan. It was strange being at a mass for my late wife and now I may have a bloody disease that may kill me. Life is horrible sometimes and I'm now thinking what do 1 do now to protect Garreth and my family. Garreth is my priority now. Suddenly I am scared of what lies ahead but I have to be brave and face it all. Work carries on as normal but everyday now I worry so much about these neck lumps.

It is November 22nd 2013 and I am now on Winter leave from work. I travelled to Razgrad to visit Milena. I met Milena while I was on holiday in Skiathos in September/October 2013. She worked in the Areti Apartments where I stayed. Anyhow I was now in Razgrad to meet all her family. On Friday November 29th I returned to Luton Airport from Varna in Bulgaria. Earlier in the day after my few days in Razgrad with Milena and her family, I drove from Razgrad to Varna Airport. Crazy Bulgarian drivers everywhere. The road from Razgrad to Varna is also the main highway between Varna and Ruse in Northern Bulgaria near the Romanian border. At night this highway is mostly in darkness. Accidents happen all the time. My flight back from Varna was a lonely one as I actually did not know when I would see Milena again. I like Razgrad but could never live there. There was a small language barrier but nothing to worry about. Anyhow I knew I would be back there as soon as possible. Milena could not travel to me as she had a son aged 11 and she was responsible for looking after her elderly mum as well. Life in Razgrad is a daily struggle. Work opportunities are almost non existing but I have no idea also how things are going to pan out for me. I will deal with things as they happen and right now I am on my way home from Bulgaria to Luton Airport. As regards my work, I was on a short period of annual leave so was glad to be home for the weekend.

On Monday December 2nd 2013, I was asked to have a PET Scan in St Thomas Hospital at 2.45pm but having nothing to eat for six hours previous to the scan time. I was scanned a little later than what was supposed to be the appointment time but it was late by only ten minutes or so. The main thing is that I was scanned. The PET Scan is a long procedure. After getting all my medication details etc, I was taken to an area that is called the hot waiting area. There after having a cannula inserted in my arm, my height and weight was noted and in the cubicle in the hot waiting area some radiation sugar is injected into my blood system via the cannula. After a wait of one and a half hours it is then expected that the radiation sugar in all that time would by now have gone into every nook and cranny in the body. I change into a hospital gown or anything really that hasn't got any metal bits like zips etc. I make my way to the scanning room and lie on a flat trolley like surface which is secured in place.

My head and neck area is scanned first over 10 to 15 minutes and then the rest of the body is scanned over another 25 minutes or so and that is it. I get dressed and return to the waiting room and as soon as the scanning machine operators are happy with the images, they come out and tell me that it is okay to leave. If anyone gets it wrong people are called in to repeat but I was allowed to go home. On Tuesday December 3rd I had to go to the Princess Royal University Hospital [PRUH] for a pre op where a biopsy was taken. I went sick from work for that. On the next day and still sick it was Wednesday December 4th 2013. I saw Dr Terry and got the results of my biopsy. I know something is not good when I noticed the medics whispering amongst each other. Dr Terry said the tests showed that I had cancer but more tests were needed. More mental agony for me and there and then I decided to go sick again from work, I cannot drive a packed bus and try not to worry about having cancer. Monday December 9th – guess what I done … yes, I went back to work to take my mind off the cancer diagnosis and, well, anyway that was the plan and the intention. Stupid move as I again went sick at work. On Friday morning, December 13th at Guys it was confirmed that I had SQUAMOUS CELL CARCINOMA of the base of the tongue. December 13th was also the Friday night where my family and I together with work colleagues all go to see the Christmas Panto in the Churchill Theatre in Bromley. Great night had by all but of course the worse bit was telling my work mates and their families. It had the same reaction just like when I was told. They are devastated.

On December 16th I saw Dr Terry in the PRUH. I do not remember the exact time but as Garreth of course knew I still had to tell Mary my sister. She was devastated and it knocked the hell out of her. Of course there is no easy way to tell your sister that you have cancer and that the end result will be death and this death would happen to me within 18 months. How the hell does anyone deal with that. I can also tell you that since that day, Mary has told me that she has every intention of calling me by phone or text but mainly by phone every single day from now on. I have no doubt that she will do this because she is in Ireland and therefore not close by and when I told her my diagnosis it did hit her ver, very hard, more so than what I expected. We have always been close but of course had our own private lives but she has always been there for me and from now on will be even more so. On the other hand it will help me enormously as having cancer is at best a very lonely place to be and worse for me as I am on my own. Of course I have Gaz my son with me night and day and he is my rock and I adore him so much, but it will be nice to have my sister Mary close by as well. I cannot thank her enough for saying this to me ... so thank you sis. I will explain later on in the book our Red and Yellow Card system between us. My brother Liam on the other hand dealt with it different and possibly may never come to terms fully with the fact that I his elder brother am going to die from bloody cancer. It happens a lot in families that other close family members cannot believe that their close loved ones are going to die and do so sooner rather than later. For all I know, I may have a similar reaction if told similar devastating news. I feel sure that he will eventually understand but I also hope that it happens before my funeral whenever that will be. In my mind right now cancer means inevitable death so it will be a shock to anyone who finds it difficult to fully accept.

On December 23rd I decided that I had to go long-term sickness because on the morning of the 23rd at Guys Hospital, I attended the Dental Clinic and had some teeth removed in advance, as a precaution because after some possible forthcoming treatment it would be better to remove teeth now rather than later. They, under the guidance of Dr M. B, then removed my 2 gold crowns. I took them home and if possible I would sell them on E-Bay. Also I went sick from work because the next day December 24th Christmas Eve I was to be in Clinic in Guys Hospital to meet Dr Theresa Guerrero-Urbano, my Consultant. By going sick from work on a long-term basis, I could then concentrate on my treatments and all the trappings of both physically and mentally dealing with the fact that I had this destructive aggressive disease called cancer. I cannot drive a bus and go through Cancer at the same time. I also knew that I could get sick certificates from my Consultant or Doctor for up to 6 months at least and possibly longer. Cancer or any disease like it is treated specially with most employers. My employer was a big named private company involved in Public Transportation. I had over twenty years service (+20 years) with this same company so long term sickness is now my only option. I will keep you all up to date of my sickness and my work but for now it is okay for me to be sick and get paid for it. I think that after 6 months my full basic pay will reduce to half pay. but that's a long way away. Do not worry my friends, things are in my favour and I have every intention of taking this as far as I can legally take it. I can also tell anyone reading this and being concerned about cancer and your job. In all the leaflets and info that are given out to cancer patients, let me tell you that it is all true and correct. Employers may try stunts and basically chance their arm. I think you could say it is dipping their elbow in the hot water to test it before jumping in.. Jump in, you have nothing to worry about because cancer patients or sufferers with the help of MacMillan and your consultant will win your rights fully. Just take the advice given to you by MacMillan etc. Even big employers like mine had a little attempt,

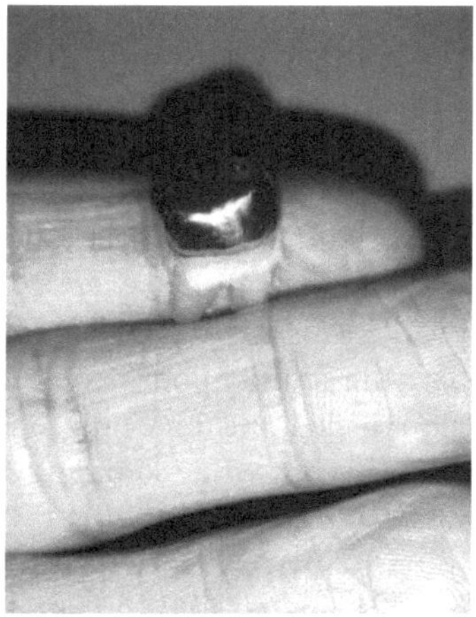

Teeth were removed in preparation for Chemo.

but failed miserably. They know also that any negative publicity can do a lot of damage and even destroy them. Long term they will not risk it. Please put your mind at ease and if I am still alive at the time this book is published, please contact me. My details will be fully available in this book. I want to help anybody who is in the same position as me. Now where was I, Oh yes! As regards my meeting with my consultant, my only child Garreth or Gaz as he is widely known was with me on this important day. I say child but he is far older than being a child, but he will always be my child. Dr Theresa Guerrero-Urbano was available and she examined me. She discovered multiple lymph nodes on the left side of my neck in levels 2, 3 and 5. The biggest one of these is 4cms x 4cms and is actually so big it is very close to breaking through the skin. My blood count was good. In the room was Dr M L and Dr P. Dr P saw me and told me the worst news ever. Dr T in The PRUH told me that they could cure me, and sure enough at the time he was right, however things have changed and Dr P told me that my cancer was no longer curable as it was now secondary and has spread to the lymph nodes in my windpipe. I had secondary cancer metastatic stage 4 and it definitely was not going to be cured. I do not know if they would tell me or not but I had to ask even though I was scared of the answer. I asked how long I had left to live, and now the reason why I do not like this. Dr P. told me that at the most I had only 12 to 18 months left to live and that it may be sooner than that. She said that they would offer me treatment but I was to understand that it is only to give me extra time if it works. However the likelihood is that it is a very aggressive cancer and the end would be quick when I was in the final stage of life.

At that moment I hated myself for having asked and my whole world fell apart. I remember bursting out crying and I buried my head in my hands. Poor Garreth who was with me put his right arm around me as if to take me under his wing. No child should have to do this and listen to a death sentence given to his parent. I feel for Garreth as he lost his mum in 2008 and now his Dad was going to die in front of him. This f*****g life is so cruel and unfair. It was Christmas eve and what a f*****g horrible present this was. I cannot remember when but my cancer nurse Hannah was in the room. I was later able to get to know Claire and Laura. They are all so kind and lovely. Theresa however, my Consultant is so, so lovely and already I think a lot of her. I did however at that very moment dislike every healthy person on this planet. Happy healthy rich people I dislike simply because I have cancer and they have not. F**k it I even hate the healthy poor people. I hate life and probably most of all I dislike Dr P who dished out my death sentence. Maybe I am feeling sorry for myself when I say this but while so many Londoners were doing their Christmas shopping I was being simply told that I was going to die and the only treatment was purely to try to give me extra time to live maybe only a matter of an extra few months on this earth. All of a sudden death seemed so soon to happen and the 18 months if I lived that long would come to an end on June 23rd 2015. At least the weather would be more than likely sunny and warm for my funeral. Dr Theresa Guerrero-Urbano is a spanish lady and she is so, so good and as I keep saying, already I think the world of her. She said that as my blood count was good they would go ahead and offer me Chemotherapy treatment. She also said if any new lumps appeared I should tell them immediately. I asked Theresa for a letter for my employers as they were harassing me a little regarding my sick spell. When I say harassing, they are being stupid and doing this to me a cancer patient is not the done thing. Employers know that there is an unwritten rule and under common decency, cancer patients are not to be rubbed up the wrong way. I have now every intention of being as normal to these employers as I can possibly be. I mean by this is that I will not go out of my way to help them. I have too much to deal with and worry about people who may mean well but they still push me about long term sickness and all such stuff. I understand that they have to do it but it is wrong and it upsets me. Theresa took a very dim view of how my employers were beginning to treat me. I knew that Theresa would keep them in line and I also spoke to MacMillan on the same matter of my nasty employers and with a combination of both MacMillan and Theresa, my employers soon stopped their "pushy attitude" and got into line. As a result, I was now in the driving seat in dealing with these people.

Let it be a warning to any employers out there, do not mess with cancer patients because you will be put in your place. I had actually seen my employers previously being nasty with sick staff and in my 20 years with the same company, I suspected that they might try something and they did, but not for long, so again employers out there, shame on you for even attempting such a stunt but ... you failed miserably. Theresa would be the one person to treat me and that was good enough. She made it clear to Gaz and I that treatment would be offered in the form of Chemotherapy or Radiotherapy or both together. She then asked Hannah my CNS to explain everything to me and that she would be guided by what I wanted to do. By that she meant if I wanted to accept the treatment or not. I cannot even accept the fact that I have cancer in the first place. Theresa wanted to see me again after a few weeks but my time off work would be at least six months but more likely to be much longer. Anyhow we had a chat and it was decided that the alternative was probably not the best as regards trying to stay alive. I now had to get through Christmas and New year. I thought of poor Garreth. What is he going to do when/if I die. Garreth is without his mum and now his Dad is going to possibly die. Eighteen months to die eh! Like I said earlier, the weather would be sunny for a June funeral. I hated the rain. I passed my bus driving test in the rain and since then I have hated the rain so please do not rain on my funeral. I want Udens in Petts Wood to do my funeral. I want everything organised before my death. Cremation in Beckenham where my Joan was cremated. I want Garreth to decide where to scatter my ashes with that of his mum. Don't mix them together as Joan would have hated that. I want to see Skiathos at least one more time or more if possible. I was learning to fly Microlights but that ended with my diagnosis. I do not want to die alone and I do not want to die in pain. There will be a white envelope prepared near the time of my end. In it are all my wishes and instructions. I realise that Chemotherapy or Radiotherapy is planned not to cure me but to buy me extra time to live for as long as possible.

——— # # # ———

CHRISTMAS DAY December 25th 2013. I had a day as good as possible with Garreth and some friends of ours. My sister Mary called as she always does every day without fail. Merry Christmas to everyone … I will write tomorrow ...

——— # # # ———

On Thursday December 26th it was arranged that I go to The Cancer Centre on the 10th floor in Guys Hospital in London. When I got there it was a guided tour of where I was to spend a lot of time receiving Chemotherapy treatment. This is where I was to have all those strange chemicals pumped into me with the one intention of keeping me alive for as long as possible. In effect Monday would for me be Infusion Day. I have stage 4 Cancer and it is spreading all over me. I have been told that my life expectancy is going to be a maximum of 18 months but it could be as little as 12 months. Anyhow today I was taken and shown around the 10th floor, reception desk and staff. The nearby waiting area was a mix of healthy looking and sick looking people. It was obvious to deduct that the sick looking people were there for the sole purpose of being treated for their cancer. The healthy looking people was where I had the problem, were they family or friends supporting the sick looking people having treatment or were they themselves in the early stages of cancer and its treatment. In the room behind was the blood testing area and it was from here that my tour began. The appointments office where I would get to know Richard, Heena and Evelyn.

I was taken down the corridor to the different Zones A B C and D. Each zone had reclining chairs maybe about 10 or more in each Zone. As I walked down accompanied by a nurse, I noticed some people were asleep and some were chatting to their family or friends that were sitting beside them. All this was totally new to me and shocked me. These poor unfortunates all had one thing in common ... yes ... they were connected up to machines. All machines making strange noises while their pumps were pumping chemotherapy chemicals into their unfortunate cancer riddled bodies. All of these patients would face many changes to their minds, their bodies and indeed their lives. The same would happen to those nearest and dearest to them. Some of these changes would change or even destroy both male and female, young and old, rich and poor. They would lose their body hair and body weight. They would suffer vomiting, tiredness, bleeding, loneliness and in many cases death, slow deaths and quick deaths. Painful deaths and painless deaths. I look at them as I walk by the zones of treatment and I wonder to myself how many of these poor cursed unfortunate souls will be alive this time next year. Some of these people and their visitors look back at me as well and probably though to themselves or for all I knew discussed amongst themselves looking at me and probably thought or said "This guy is new"and I wonder will I be actually alive this time next year. Cancer sufferers are a strange type of f*****g breed of human being. Brave people we are, but also very unfortunate that we have been selected by cancer to join in this lottery of life and death. In this lottery of being selected to have cancer, the treatment is both painful and horrible, so painful and horrible that sufferers consider themselves winners when death releases them from their earthly agony. Cancer turns people into piles of human debris.

As I walk down further I can hear the chemotherapy infusion machines whirring away and some even bleeping. It was all completely new to me and I would soon learn their various noises. The bleeping noise is when a bag of chemotherapy or accompanied infusion chemicals like Piriton or Saline has emptied or when there is a kink in the tube and the flow has suddenly stopped. I also noticed some patients wearing headgear that makes them look like jockeys. I was told after I asked that these helmets are specially for people who wear them as cold water circulates around their heads when wearing these helmets. Apparently it helps patients not to lose their hair in chemotherapy, however it was not for me as I am already a follicly challenged human being, basically I am bald. A lot is going on here. In some cases it means that the patient with the bleeping machine, can be a patient that has finished for the day or in some cases their treatment has ended for the immediate future until it is needed again. This place is mad and busy.

The tour was soon over and I was asked to return the next day on December 27th. I done so and in the same place on the 10th floor, I was introduced to Ernie. Ernie, in normal day to day living, is the name of the machine that selects the numbers of winning Premium Bonds. This Ernie was different, it was a male nurse in the Cancer Day Unit who fits cancer patients with PICC Lines. These lines are done by ultrasound and they are the tubes put in the upper arms into a blood vessel and into which a cannula is fitted that connects up the liquid chemotherapy by infusion. This line has to be fitted properly as it uses the human heart to suck in and pump the chemotherapy around the blood system in the body. Because of the speed of the blood flow and where the blood goes to, no part of the body is missed out. Nobody left that room until the job was done properly and all the handiwork was all wrapped up in a dressing and a covering. I also knew that as I left that room the next big thing for me is chemotherapy. It was all very scary for me as it is my first time. So many things are now happening to me that I never though would happen but this is what has been given to me as part of my life. I don't want it but no going back now. I don't feel sick at all but my consultant tells me that I am very sick and my cancer is Head and Neck Cancer. It is an aggressive one and my outcome is death. Mad or what, I am doing all this chemotherapy and in the end I may die. My day was over for today in this place. I met everyone that I was suppose to meet. Ernie certainly has a big responsible job to get it in the correct position. It's a strange feeling but in a matter of days I start my chemo treatment. The idea is that the chemotherapy kills all the cells good and bad but then the good cells recover. It's a chance that I have to take but I will explain more on the day of treatment. I left and made my way to the ground floor It was late in the day and everyone had the same idea and to get home. However I sat down in the coffee area in Guys and just watched people rushing about. It's strange even here. Because it's a hospital, if you look sick or of a strange appearance nobody takes a second glance.

Outside in the front of the entrance it's the same. As soon as you reach the pavement boundary of the hospital, people look on you as if you have a walking disease. I decided to get my ass in gear and go home. It was rush hour in London Bridge and the train would be packed. I had to get home and think more of what the future held for me. The train journey as expected was a nightmare. I had walked to the far end of the platform as the station was undergoing refurbishment in part and this end was the quietest and as the time would progress in the future I would recognise faces according to the time of the day. I wonder if there was any cancer patients amongst us all on the train queue. Getting on the train was hell but I got on it. Today I was strong and not needing a seat but in future as I got weaker I would need a seat. I would eventually get to know the staff in Orpington Station like Peter and Roxy. I got home and as I shut the door behind me, I thought there is no going back now. I had cancer and there's no going back now, it's just my bad luck, many people survive it, but many do not. I can always remember reading or hearing about someone "he's fighting cancer", so this suddenly was to be me. People would now be planning to say "Oh David Cosgrave, he's fighting cancer". Now I was a statistic, a cancer sufferer. Very soon I would start my treatment, have no idea what a ride it's going to be or if I would be alive at the end of it all or even how I would look.

——— # # # ———

Hi all It is December 28th. Saturday today and mentally I feel bad. Physically I feel okay but I am counting the days down to treatment day. Sorry, no more today, God Bless and tomorrow I write more.

——— # # # ———

Sunday December 29th ... This morning I went to 10am mass in my church at St Swithun's in Fashoda Rd, Bromley Common. Before and after the mass I had to tell so many people that my cancer was being treated with chemotherapy. I am a Catholic so I want my God to take it away or let me die. I have to accept what is planned for me. Sunday is a day that nobody does anything. Some go to church and some do not. For me it's a day just wondering how the hell and why did I get cancer. I will probably think this until the day that I die, then for me it will be over, but for those I left behind, they are alive at the end of it and how would I look. Well here goes, in the meantime it's the phone calls. Mary my sister called as usual. Phone calls from so many people feeling sorry for me and so many not feeling sorry for me but still pretending by saying the nice words. This is where I start weeding out the fakes. Many of these people who say the words "feeling sorry" but actually couldn't care less one way or the other because their lives are so busy that "it's nice to be nice". Their niceness doesn't last long but in reality they are too busy. All this and it's only in the first couple of f*****g days. I haven't started my treatment yet and they have already done their bit. Anyhow that's the last I would hear from them for at least a week or so. A week is about the time limit of their fake pretence. They never fail to amuse me and they always do it. This week allows them to carry on with their life and with my sickness a week is about right for them to call me again. God only knows how my serious sickness has got in the way of their normal day to day living. The funny thing is that I would never get a visit from most of these fakes so a phone call is about their limit of contact. They do not know that I am ahead of them and weeded them out. Fakes come in all shapes, sizes and even from my family, not close family but yes within the family connections. They will never change unless maybe they have the bad luck to get cancer or a life changing sickness or accident, then maybe they will see the error of their ways. It is a very, very lonely place to be fighting cancer on your own, yes fighting. Already I am fighting, fighting the disease, fighting the health system and fighting to keep ahead of those who pretend to care for me. It's all about fighting, not physically fighting but you know what I mean. Anyhow lets see what tomorrow brings. Good Day to all of you.

——— # # # ———

It is Monday December 30th 2013 and I have nothing really to add here, except to say the mind games are active. Sorry, but I will try to write tomorrow on New Years Eve.

——— # # # ———

Tomorrow. Tuesday December 31st 2013. Well it's New Years Eve, a time to celebrate getting the old year out of the way and welcoming in the New Year and looking forward to that New Year. The calls started, Happy New Year to one and all. Happy New Year to my sister and brother and their families in Ireland. As usual I had a nice chat with Mary as what I do every day. The other phone calls started with "hello Dave, how are you", I am already thinking "How do you think I am". I am a statistic. I am now a person who has the Big C. Yes the Big C, Cancer is a terrible disease. It destroys people. It destroys families. It destroys lifestyles. It kills young and old. It kills males and females. It creates inheritances. It controls the populations in countries. It kills Kings and Queens, Princes and Princesses. It kills Presidents, Prime Ministers, newsreaders. It even kills journalists who do programmes on the bloody disease. It kills all living creatures on this planet Earth. It has no respect for the body that it invades, kills the cells, kills the person and simply moves on to the next victim. There is no way to stop it in it's path of destruction. Now let's go back to the question about how am I, I simply reply that I am okay and then I carry on with a normal conversation. Of course the fakes love my reply that I am okay, then they are happy and move on. You know what, I have never phoned anyone who was about to face chemotherapy after getting the cancer diagnosis.. It's still morning and the house is clean. I suppose that housework is the last thing on anybody's mind facing cancer treatment but tomorrow is my last normal day of living before my Chemotherapy on the 2nd. Life is all about survival of the fittest. Right now I am sitting in my conservatory doing this writing of my life. I have to fight to live and right now it's a bit like where I am right now. A small bee has become trapped in a small spider web and I can hear it squealing and like me fighting for it's life. His fight is futile as beside him is the spider who created that web with the intention of catching the bee. This poor unfortunate bee is well and truly f****d. His future is over but at this stage my future and that of the bee changes. The death of the bee is imminent, probably a few minutes. When I die, I am certainly not coming back as a bee ... before I carry on, the bee just died.. so many problems in my mind. And this is my position.

If Theresa is right, then this year ahead for me is going to be a pretty rough one. I had a chat with Gaz and I told him nothing changes. Gaz had plans to go out with his mates for months and months. My diagnosis is only a matter of weeks old then of course he has a life as well. As for me and what I learned this past 24 hours I had better get used to the idea of next Christmas and New Year being my last one, I would be a barrel of laughs out tonight. Can you imagine Happy New year everyone and by the way after next Christmas, I won't be celebrating anymore cos I am going to die. So on this December 31st I was at home alone and I cried and cried most of the evening. As Big Ben struck midnight in London I watched it on the TV. Gaz was busy with his mates but he still took time to call me and we wished each other all the very best for 2014.

However we both knew that all of 2014 would be taken up with my cancer, its treatment and any consequences. Anyhow Gaz carried on with his evening and night and I was so glad that he did exactly that. I was going to spend my time at home. I celebrated New Year but it was less exciting. I was on Facebook messenger to Milena who was working in Hotel Mimosa in Razgrad. At least that is what she told me. Who knows, but one thing I know is that is if she is working or not, and for all I know she may be cheating on me. I can do nothing about it but cry, think and worry about the future for me in 2014. My main job now is to live as long as possible, not if but for how long. My last memory of 2013 was earlier in the day of the 31st I had to endure a camera down my throat via my right nostril. It was painful and made me choke but had to be done, yes will not forget my last painful memory of 2014. After the Fireworks etc on telly was over, I did actually chat to Milena online for a while. Then I went to bed and just wanted to put 2013 behind me and wake up in 2014.

——— # # # ———

January 1st New Years Day was just crap. I had gone into a New Year with many problems. 'Let me explain … I got myself into New YEAR and Here I am on the first day of 2014. I attended Guys Hospital in London for an appointment to meet Dr P after an early morning call to come up. and the rest of the team that are now taking care of me. I would take a dislike to this woman for what she was going to say and confirm to me. It's a bloody weird thing but when you are called into a room to see the results of a medical scan or examination. If there is one person in the room to see you, you get the feeling that it may not be too bad. However if there is more than one or two then you get that bad anxious feeling in the pit of your stomach that maybe the news is probably not too good. Today, January 1st was basically confirmation before treatment goes ahead tomorrow. In the room waiting for me was a group, a hit squad, not good as bad news it was too. Apart from Dr P. also present was Hannah my CNS, My speech and language therapist, my dietician, my physiotherapist and occupational therapist. It was also explained to me that as my cancer is so aggressive my chemo treatment will be severe. Chemotherapy treatment will start tomorrow, January 2nd, and it will be in 6 cycles with each cycle lasting 3 weeks. Therefore it will be over a period of over 18 weeks if all goes smoothly and to plan. Week 1 is over a period of 6 hours or so, I will have infusion of CISPLATIN and then 5FU and sent home with a pump full of 5FU going in 24/7 for 4 days before disconnection by a District nurse who comes out to my home ... Week 2 vis over a period of about 3 to 4 hours infusion of 5FU and then home followed by Week 3 and over a period of 3 to 4 hours again more 5FU and home. That is the plan anyway. Nothing of course ever goes to plan and my treatment was no exception. Dr P never done me harm but what she told me would destroy the remainder of my life of course no fault to her but she was only doing her job. Of course she again said those important but horrible words "I am sorry David but..." Once I heard those words I knew the rest was bad. She confirmed again that my cancer was no longer curable and I am now to have Palliative care eventually leading to end of life. I had metastatic disease of a squamous cell carcinoma. I was devastated, why me? How was it me? How did it happen to me? What did I ever do wrong in life to get punished like this. I asked her what was next and then burst into tears and screamed out loud. I cried and cried and cried and cried. Again I hated all healthy people in the world. I left and went into a nearby room with Hannah my CNS. Poor Garreth ... but we both decided to do as much as possible to live as long as possible ... How can my brain take in the fact that I am supposed to die in 12 to 18 months. Terminal Cancer means death. My next birthday is 57th and it may be my last and I probably will have one more Christmas. As I said before, I want Udens in Petts Wood to do my funeral. Speak to Len there and I like flowers. Okay tomorrow is treatment day. Let's try and beat that eighteen months deadline. I have no idea what to expect...

——— # # # ———

JANUARY 2nd 2014 ... Good morning all, big day today. I have to get the train to London Bridge from Orpington. Maybe it will be easier than expected, I don't know, but lets see. I got off at London Bridge Station. On the short trip from Orpington, my mind was blank. Earlier I got chatting to Peter one of the platform staff in Orpington. I was to get to know very well Peter, Roxy and Simon. In London Bridge I walked down the ramp from the platform, down the escalator and turned left past the arcade of shops. Everybody was rushing about and I was thinking how many of them had cancer and not even knew about it. I also though how many of them had personal private battles in their own lives. They may be okay for now but more and more people are getting cancer so to be totally honest, their future is not as rosy as it appears now. The curse of cancer is more real than what it appears. They however may be lucky enough to have so many more treatments than what is available now. Anyhow I made my way towards Guys Hospital, I walked past MacDonalds and the beggars on the steps. I thought would it be better to be a healthy beggar or be like me as a cursed cancer sufferer. Yes it is a curse if you get cancer and me, well I am well cursed. I have the terminal cancer, the type that is one day going to kill me. The hospital say that I will be dead in 18 months, but my big trick is to prove them wrong.

Anyhow, I got to the corner of Guys turned left past the smoking patients in pyjamas and a drip trolley and a lighted cigarette in the other hand, bloody joke it is. In I go through the revolving doors that people run to beat and it jams to a halt and everybody is delayed by the careless actions of one idiot who thought it was a good idea at the time to beat the revolving door. I made my way past the queue for the coffee at AMT with all the doctors and nurses queuing up. I thought there must be nobody on the bloody wards. Anyhow my destination was the Cancer Day Unit on the 10th floor. I got into the lift and pressed 10 and I was on my way. I got to the 10th floor and stepped out. Different world up here I thought. So many people have taken this lift day after day and are no longer with us and I expect that there are many people who have survived but would be in their graves was it not for the Cancer Day Unit and its staff and doctors etc. I am heading up the corridor through the double doors and there I was at the reception desk. Another queue awaited me. When the time came I presented my appointment booklet and had a wristband put on my wrist like I was all inclusive on holiday. On that wristband was my name and hospital number 5*****6T and my date of birth. I took a seat in the nearby waiting room and we done what waiting rooms are there for, we waited. I looked around me and straight away noticed the sick, haggard looking people, tired, worn and bedraggled. These were the scariest, sickest, unfortunate people that I ever did see. My God these people were ill and I thought that one day soon after a few treatments that I am going to look like them and then any new people coming in for the first time will look at me and think that I look like sick, tired, worn, bedraggled, haggard and very ill. For the moment I looked healthy and resembled some of the other people sitting down. Some of these healthy people were family or friends of sick people or like me were to be future patients. For now I am okay but that would soon change. At the reception desk was Richard and Evelyn dishing out the ID Wristbands.

In the office nearby was Heena. I would get to know these people very well in the next few months. Anyhow my name was called by a cancer nurse who had come from the treatment area to the waiting room. We both walked back down to the treatment area and into one of the zones. I forget which zone I was in but anyhow I was shown to a seat. All the seats were Recliner so I sat in my already allocated Recliner. It was in the corner as there you can see all that goes on all around. I looked around as that is where the sick and dying are separated from the healthy and living. If you are a patient you are guaranteed to be in a recliner but this the limit of the comfort for the day. This was to be my home from home for the next 6 hours or so. It's a God forsaken place but it is comfortable, warm and spotless and in the recliners you get a blanket and a pillow. As I already had a PICC line in my left upper arm I was soon the centre of attention as one of the nurses pushed a trolley in my direction with all its medical gear requirements on it including swabs, tissues, tubes, plasters and cotton wool. Underneath that had more shelves with further items needed in the department. I was then told that treatment would begin soon. I had no idea as everything was totally new to me. If they had told me that it would start in a few hours, well was okay by me as I had no idea at all. Two nurses stood over me, One to sign for the treatment and the other to witness the first signature of the nurse setting up and connecting me to the chemotherapy treatment packs which were soon to be on their way into me and beginning my fight back to stay alive for as long as possible. The PICC line is located and the tubes are connected. Here we go as it begins its journey into my body and around inside me. No going back now. Piriton was one of the first packs of treatment that was put into me and it would make me drowsy and thus send me off to sleep. This was followed by bags of saline at intervals. Between the intervals were the remaining chemotherapy treatments of Cisplatin and 5FU. I looked around me and everything fascinated me now. Bleeping noises all around, nurses in plastic disposable aprons. Nurses with disposable rubber gloves running about everywhere. These nurses are angels and everyone is treated with so much unconditional love, respect, dignity and care.

This is my first day, my first few hours, I knew nothing yet. Around me everyone is in the same f****** mess, we are all diseased with Cancer. Some of us will be cured, some of us will get a little bit of remission but sadly so many of us will die. In my case I have been told first of all that it was curable but then I was told that I am to ultimately die in 18 months or less from now. I may get a small amount of remission but the end story for me is death. My story therefore in the end is destined to eventually not have a happy ending. Not one of us including me, knows the exact day when we will die but it will happen. Another thing I noticed today is as I noticed the day I had my tour of this place is that there are some patients in their seats resembling jockeys wearing helmets on their heads and as I already mentioned is a device with cold water running through it to prevent any hair loss during chemotherapy. With cancer, chemotherapy and hair loss go side by side. Anyhow it's time for me to sleep in my recliner, I was drifting off to sleep and I can't fight it anymore and have no intention of fighting off sleep anymore. I later woke up with someone poking me. It was Lucy, one of the nurses asking me to confirm my date of birth as some drugs were being administered to me. I had to be awake for this one. PICC line located and Cisplatin was first in after the Piriton over a time of less than two hours. I am now thinking my body must be going through hell as it has never known before these drugs going into it. All for the first time. It's strange but all these cancer drugs of chemotherapy that I am getting are clear liquids but they are expected to do me some good. My cancer has an outward appearance of massive lumps in my neck. These lumps were my Lymph glands swelled into action by the cancer, Head and Neck Cancer but also now had gone secondary into my windpipe. It would take a lot of Chemo to sort this one out and change things around. I have no idea how all this one is going to pan out. Another thing I noticed is that all the chemotherapy bags on drip going into me and every bag of Chemotherapy is protected from the light by a darker coloured plastic bags and in my case it was mainly blue plastic bags that covered my chemotherapy packs. Anyhow, I am still in my recliner, feet up and getting sleepy again despite all the bleeping noises all around me. It is so lovely and warm here. I was to get used to all this. As I said earlier my treatment is palliative care, no cure for me, but I do believe in miracles! My diagnosis of the cancer is such that mine is stage 4 so it's quite late and therefore my treatment is solely to buy me time to try to live for as long. I will take whatever they give me in treatment but what they give me at this stage has to be aggressive as otherwise a mild lesser dose of treatment may not be enough to have any effect on my cancer. Gaz came in to see me on his break from work Bless him, He had hopped on a bus and of course it was lovely to see him but he has to look after his job too. Jobs do not grow on trees and after I have passed away he will need his job. He did not deserve this worry of me getting cancer. He is however taking it well but his girlfriend by his side helps I hope. I think a lot of her and that may be because if I pass away, I would love it he had someone in his life and I would not worry about him being alone after I die. Maybe I am silly but most dads probably think the same way. Anyhow Gaz had to go back to work. I must have nodded off to sleep because soon I am being woken up by the nurses asking me my details again etc.

This time the 5FU Chemotherapy pack is being connected up and infused into me and then covered over by a red bag to block out any light getting at it. The snacks trolley comes around and I had tea and a sandwich. I loved it all and soon I was feeling sleepy again. Looking around me, I noticed that more new people were in the other recliner seats. I thought, My God, people are coming and going here at a fast rate. It is so busy. Visitors coming and going here and I still haven't got into a conversation with anyone of them. My appointment was at 08.30 this morning and it's now a little after 2.15pm and am into my second and final chemotherapy of the day. This one as I said is 5FU and is also the one that I will have going home in a pump connected up to me 24/7. As I said before the nurses approach me in pairs and then after checking between them the correct details of the chemotherapy pack. Inn all cases everything is double checked. No mistakes here, all very professional and all carried out like clockwork precision. My time here today would soon be over. I am staying awake now as I don't want to miss any important bits. I do not feel any different as yet but it is early days and I have only had a couple of bags of chemotherapy going around inside me. The fight back has started. My thinking is that there is no way they would give me something unless it might do some good to me. I was disconnected from my machine. Around me the noises continued of other patients who of course were having their treatments of their own very private battles and fightback with their cancer. Other voices were nurses talking to other nurses and other patients. All of us in here on the 10th Floor in Guys have one thing in common, we are all after being handed a potential death sentence and we are all fighting back with the help of bags of chemicals that have given us a small promise of cheating death. Death does not like been cheated out of its intention and therefore as a result some of us will die and some of us will live ... for a while longer. Eventually death wins in the end and will always get its way with or without cancer to make its intention a little easier. Anyhow as I still looked around the patients that had the headgear resembling jockeys were still here, well saying that I only noticed the three patients with that headgear in my immediate vicinity of the zone that I was in. I for one did not opt for any of these chemo caps because I was already challenged in the follicle department and as a result had no hair to be protected anyway. After I was disconnected from the machine, I was then connected to my lovely Chemo Pump and with various straps attached to the Pump Unit which were then attached to me by wearing them across my shoulder from top left shoulder to right waist area, the pump and its sealed contents of 5FU would then be going into me 24/7 over the next 4 days. I collected my appointment card and left the 10th floor area and got into the lift and pressed G.

My next destination was simply the ground floor of Guys Hospital. My little blue appointment booklet was looking so sorrowful with very few appointments in it, but it would soon fill up. I was now permanently attached to my Chemo pump pack. I was going to do every damn thing in the world in this outfit. It was connected to my bloodstream and as it was attached to me, It therefore went everywhere with me and whatever I done. As I left the hospital I did feel weird. By looking at me from the outside, nobody could tell but inside my clothes was this chemo unit hidden from view.. I made my way past McDonalds and crossed the road towards the Shard, past the guy giving out the Evening Standard paper, up the escalator past the security staff for the Shard across the forecourt of the entrance to Southern Trains nearly getting blown away because every time I go up this area it seems to always blow a gale. Today this open space was both windy and bloody freezing. I made my way into London Bridge Station and onto the platform to get the train to Orpington. I felt okay now but the chemo would take effect in a couple of days especially when the attached pump would start to empty itself into by bloodstream. Anyhow I got home and indoors. I reckon the fun would really begin in earnest in the morning when I would try and shower. It is now Monday evening going into night. A district nurse would come out to me in 4 days time to disconnect the chemo pump from my PICC line and clean the area around it. Tomorrow morning is Friday. I have had enough of today, too much has happened and it is really a lot to take in. All new to me and all very, very strange. Goodnight all and may your God Bless you all. Goodbye to Thursday January 2nd 2014. I was stuck with a pump all weekend pumping chemo 5FU into me until disconnection sometime Monday evening or Monday night.

——— # # # ———

Good Morning all it's Friday JANUARY 3rd 2014. I have had a really shit night trying to sleep with this f****** pump. Inside this pump unit is a little sealed window and looking in I can see a balloon full of clear chemotherapy liquid and already I can see it shrinking a little. My actual treatment which I believe I have already said is Chemotherapy infusion only in 6 cycles with each cycle being 3 weeks, therefore a total of about 18 weeks. The chemotherapy is in WEEK 1 CISPLATIN, 5FU ALL INFUSED OVER ABOUT 6 HOURS IN GUYS HOSPITAL AND A PUMP OF 5FU AT HOME OVER 4 DAYS AND 24/7. WEEK 2 5FU INFUSION OVER 3 HOURS IN GUYS HOSPITAL AND WEEK 3 5FU AGAIN INFUSION OVER 3 HOURS IN GUYS HOSPITAL... TOTAL THEREFORE FOR 1st CYCLE OF TREATMENT IS ABOVE. TOTAL CYCLES IS EXPECTED 6 CYCLES ALL OVER 18 WEEKS, BUT IS ALL LIABLE TO ALTERATION AT SHORT NOTICE .... It's a long way away to 4 months and 2 weeks. Anyhow going back to the shower from hell this morning, the plan was and will be to keep the PICC Line and the pump dry, a tall request but got to be done. It is therefore a very, very slow process to shower properly. It was done but it took over 45 minutes.

The weekend is almost here and am now eagerly awaiting Monday night and the district nurse visiting and disconnecting the pump. I have no idea how my body is reacting to these chemicals going in to me. My body like any body has never experienced chemotherapy ever before. Chemicals that someone clever and responsible has put together specially for me based on what they know of me and my cancer diagnosis. I am thinking, how in the name of God am I to take this persons decision that this batch of Chemotherapy Liquid is good and correct for me. Racist thinking goes out the window in this situation. I have no idea what nationality or religious belief is the person or persons that put my bags of chemotherapy together, nor do I care as long as it gives me a chance to live a little longer. We all know that cancer has no rules. It just makes people very sick and then it kills them. It kills all creeds, ages, sexes and colours. I have no idea what will happen but I do know what is happening to me now. The outcome of the next eighteen weeks may have interesting results. Chemotherapy has failed many people but it has also saved many others. This is my 1st week of Chemotherapy. Look at me now, all you can see is a large cluster of lumps on my neck. No other outward signs of cancer. However, cancer does take many forms. In all, I am facing around 120 days of chemotherapy. I look okay now but that will soon change as both the cancer and the chemo battle it out on my body. They couldn't care less as both of them want to win but we know there is only one winner.

With the treatment I have to get sick to get better. I am facing Hair loss, ingrowing toe nails, weight loss, random vomiting, bleeding from any part of the body that decides to bleed on any random day of the week for no reason whatsoever. I am facing my body feeling cold and tired. I will have blankets and hot water bottles yet still facing shivering and tiredness. I will be wiped clean of energy, I will struggle to walk and maybe struggle to talk. I am facing food and drinks having a horrible metallic or cardboard taste. I will have a body rash but my face will be very badly affected. Therefore, I will go through pure hell when shaving. All of these reactions are already in the paperwork as being the most likely reactions to the two Chemotherapy treatments that I am having pumped into me, well lets see. It scares me because I do not doubt for one minute that the information leaflets are wrong. Today Friday January 3rd 2014 is nearly over. Lets see if the experts are actually correct. Time for a cuppa before I lose the taste of tea. For now no metal etc taste but give it time, it will soon happen. Maybe tomorrow will be the same as today. Good night all.

——— # # # ———

GOOD MORNING ALL, it's Saturday January 4th 2014. Had a shower after a poor night of sleep. Getting used to the showering part of the day but it is still awkward taking a shower. The balloon of chemo is now gone down a little, that only means one thing. Yes, the chemo is inside me and doing its work on my cancer, I hope. It's Day 2, it's Saturday and the first thing I look at every day is the balloon of Chemotherapy. I can't ignore it, I sleep with the damn thing. I wear the support straps of this pump across my chest from left to right sideways, left shoulder to right waist. I say pump but maybe pump is wrong word as the pump is actually my heart via my PICC Line sucking the chemo into my bloodstream. This bloody pump, I do everything in it, toilet, shower, walking, driving, eating, drinking and sleeping. I can't imagine sex is fun wearing one of these. I am sure it's the same with anyone with one of these pumps that sex in any form is out of the question in Week 1 of every cycle of this type of treatment. I won't dwell on this matter but you can imagine how it's done and still wearing a bulky item like this balloon full of chemotherapy. I dare say some people bypass the problems but I can assure you that if you can go without this form of pleasure in your life, then by all means go without. It's a much more "easy way out" if you can do without. I can tell you one thing that crosses my mind very regularly and it's bloody scary, it's a burning question which is this, "what if they got my diagnosis wrong" and now all these chemicals are going into my body and what if they are not needed for the cancer, what damage are they doing. I have one answer for that, I have to believe that the experts have got it right and the treatment is correct. This is the only answer that I can believe in. If I think otherwise then it will tear me apart and destroy me. They are the consultants and I am the patient and that is the way it's going to be until the day I die. If the cancer has its way then in 18 months from now I will be either dead or in a hospice dying. If it works then I will have my way and have bought extra time and still be alive and kicking and maybe enjoying life in one way or another. Soon, however, I will be looking like shit. They are the bosses and they control my life now. Tomorrow is Sunday January 5th and for today I have nothing further to add. The rest of today is normal for me. I will write again tomorrow. In a way I am looking forward to tomorrow. It's my last full balloon day. The balloon of chemotherapy is deflating now every day but today seems full, even though the District Nurse is due tomorrow. This balloon, however, looks too full for disconnection tomorrow, like it has more life in it than I expect. Tonight I have just noticed that I am feeling cold and tired. Could it be happening already, I suppose it might be. Goodnight all. I write again tomorrow.

——— # # # ———

Hi all, it's Sunday January 5th 2014. Good Morning and as it is a Sunday, I think I am going to mass today for 10am and I feel good apart from being very tired, more tired than usual. The pump and balloon however looks very full and if the district nurse arrives, she will be going away to come back again tomorrow. She decides when to come out, so no point in me contacting her to cancel. However, I have now decided not to go to mass for three reasons. I cannot take the chance of missing that district nurse visiting and the other two reasons, the sheer physical inability because of that stupid annoying but essential chemo pump and balloon. Since January 2nd my blood is now mixed with lovely chemotherapy. My blood is now useless to anyone else but me alone because of it being contaminated but I can take donations of AB+ blood group. Therefore the other reason is Mass and why I cannot attend. The pump is the main reason but if I go to mass I get something like a bag of liquorice all sorts, a mixture of everyone. The genuine people and the nosey f*****s. The genuine people are exactly that, they do well and they mean well. However it's the nosey f*****s that have only one purpose in life and that is to pry into the lives of other people and other people's business. If I had gone to mass today, the nosey fu****s would be on duty just to ask me questions on my cancer, the treatment and how it is affecting me, my family and friends. Then, if these nosey bastards do not get the answers that they were expecting, they would add their little bit to make it seem more interesting and then spread the gossip, idle gossip. They are also the same ones that sit at the back of the church in their prime locations. They even get to the church early just to get these exclusive seating arrangements. My god, these people treat these seats like season ticket seat holders at Old Trafford, The Emirates or Stamford Bridge. To them, these prime seats are like gold dust. They forget the sole reason in church is to pray and seek forgiveness for their wrongdoing in their day-to-day living. If they sat at the front or half way up they are ruined, scarred for life simply because they cannot see or control over what they see or who they see coming into the church, but at the back of the church, WOW WOW! They can see everything in who to plan their "attack" on and "approach" their "target" for a bout of nosey questioning. Today I would have been that target. So ... NO! They can remain in their prime location season ticket church seats and select another poor unfortunate victim of circumstances. At 9am I changed my mind and went to mass. I took a chance that the district nurse would not come to me early in the day. My God won in the end and I need mass now whenever I can, if I can. I met people after Mass both the genuine people and the fakes. I spent most of the time chatting to the genuine people at this morning's mass. I spoke to the fakes too but they hovered over my shoulder and listened in to my normal conversation with the genuine people. Like I said before, the fakes have already decided for themselves what news I had to tell and then they decide for themselves if it suits their agenda or not and of course if not they just add to what they already know. People are strange, these fakes are strange.

I came home from Mass but thinking back I had a good chat with Mary S, Sandra C and Mark, Pearl, Monica, John and Jackie and my good lovely friend Anne who lost her husband some time ago. Anne, John and Jackie and I always sit side by side in the same seat in our Church. John always sits on the aisle end of seat and when the priest goes wild with the holy water blessing everyone supposedly, but actually soaking everyone, poor John is a glutton for punishment and gets splashed on his spectacles every time. However he never changes his mind to move seats. One day soon, I can see people coming to these masses and any other church ceremonies with a change of clothes depending on which priest is on doing any holy water blessings. Away from the Church, I phone my friend Anne from time to time and as I said, we are really good friends. These are all the most honest sincere genuine people anyone could meet and I am pleased to call them genuine friends. The "fakes" who listened nearby are the people who pretend to care but in reality they couldn't give a toss about anyone but themselves. Yes, the fakes are all around us even in my family, distant family but still classed as family. It is hard to believe but I hope to be brave enough to expose the fakes in this book. They know who they are because they have been fakes all of their lives. Once a fake, always a fake. Fakes, crooks the lot of them, they will all burn in hell where they have places already allocated and waiting for them. In the meantime it carries on, though some have retired and they know who they are, so when they read their headline in my book they may be shocked to read about the strange fact that all along I knew they were"fakes". Now it is I who has had the last laugh because those fakes etc were never aware that I knew all along how cheap and false they were and I played along to your every move but was actually one step ahead of you all along. Another fake bound for the flames of eternal fire in hell, ha ha! They will not drag me down. I am in enough shit with this cancer, so it's time to try to get better now that I have had my moment of fun.

Moving on, my gastric band which I have had since 2009 and over 24 stone and 3 lbs is still a little restricted but worked a treat as I am now just over 12 stone, so no great eating today. I feel for my only child Garreth, but he is being so strong for me about all this. He is my tower of strength right now but we have to be strong for each other as it will all get far worse before it gets better, or if it gets better. The District nurse came out at 5.15pm this evening but, as expected, she left just as quick to return tomorrow. The balloon had a lot of chemo in it and of course she had to make the decision to disconnect or not and disconnecting was not in my benefit right now I still had the benefit of getting all the chemo in that pump. Is it having any effect? Yes it is, in that already I feel very tired now always and all the lumps in my neck which totalled 12 or 14 seem to have stopped getting any bigger. I feel different and it is only a bloody week. Lets see tomorrow when it's disconnected. For some reason now I want to get every drop of this chemotherapy liquid. I don't want to die. Bring it on now! No going back now!

Okay, that is it for today. I have had my daily phone call from Mary, my sister. I may not mention it every day, but I can assure you we do speak every day. Bless her for doing this and keep an eye on me, as does Gaz of course. Another thing is that I may refer to Gaz as my only child. He is in his 20's but as far as I am concerned he is still my child. Tomorrow is Monday, January 6th and a new day. Will I feel and look any different tomorrow? Who knows! Goodnight all. God Bless you all.

——— # # # ———

Morning all. It's Monday January 6th. I am tired like I said and cold but no other differences in my condition. Looking down now at the pump and balloon of chemotherapy, I am glad to say that it's nearly empty of chemo liquid. That can only mean one thing, its all gone into me. The District nurse is due back here later on tonight or this evening. I have also been injecting myself in the belly with Clexane for blood thinning. I have lovely bruising in the belly now as a result of this. The day progressed as normal as possible. Showered as normal as possible with the pump and try not getting anything too wet as a result. I had covered the area of the PICC Line with cling film to keep out the water. What a waste of time that was. The District nurse came at 4.45pm. She disconnected the pump unit and disposed of it in a sharps bin, same bin as my Clexane Blood thinning needles. She then disinfected and cleaned the entire area and dressed it for my next chemo connection and infusion appointment in Guys Cancer Day Unit. Before leaving me, she made her report and left a copy with me. She has done very little as regards my disconnection etc so not much of a report to write, so am glad that very little ink was used for the report. Can't blame me for any excess use of ink then. What a relief to be free of that bloody pump and no idea yet when next chemo session of Week 2 Cycle 1 is going to be. From what I understand they are giving me a small break already so my system gets used to the treatment, so no idea as yet when next one is. The Lymph glands where the cancer is are now sticking out of my neck like massive lumps on the side of my neck all around now nearly. This Head and Neck cancer is now spreading. It is very aggressive and soon my neck will be full of lumps all around. Unless this is stopped it will kill me soon, so bring on the next chemotherapy as quickly as possible. The rest of today is just thinking and wondering "what if". It bothers me now, every minute of the day, why I have been cursed with cancer. I cry now daily, and it's hitting me that I will die from this disease. I cry and cry and cry and cry, me a grown man crying. Nothing to do now but go to bed crying myself to sleep. No pump tonight and I will sleep well and turn and twist without restrictions of a chemo pump. However, it's hitting me, I'm dying, slowly dying, Goodnight all. Tomorrow is Tuesday January 7th, a new day.

——— # # # ———

Hi all, yes it is a new day. I want to stay in bed, I am so, so bloody tired, drained of all energy. Nowadays there is nothing to do at home but think, think of what I have done and thinking ahead of what I may be doing as things progress. I was always told as a kid that thinking is dangerous because you never get what you want anyway. The sun is low in the sky today and the day is short. It is dark for a long time now, from night to near 7am and again at 3.30pm the darkness returns. Winter is a lonely depressing feast of months and as a result I just do a lot of thinking and sleeping day in and day out. As far as I am concerned, the longer I sleep, the less I have to think and worry about my cancer. I cry now randomly, It has hit me so hard that I am actually dying. It is something that I cannot get out of my mind. I can't hide from it. The grim reaper has selected me and is coming in my direction. I am going to die early in my life and nobody can do anything about it. Darkness is my daily saviour but my God as soon as daylight begins to reappear, my pain and torment resumes. Yes, pain and torment resumes. Now I am looking for a calendar with the various times of dawn and sunset but no calendar to hand to help me work out my times of when it is actually dark, where I can then know when I can get my most peace, rest and also not thinking. Like I said, I treasure the hours of darkness, I'm sure Dracula had the same idea of making the most of darkness but unlike him, I sleep and do not think or worry about the future that lies ahead. Tomorrow is Wednesday January 8th and I have to see My consultant Theresa Guerrero-Urbano or a member of her team. I have no idea why they need to see me … Goodnight all.

——— # # # ———

Hi all, it is Wednesday January 8th 2104 and my consultant appointment in Guys is at 1pm. I did some housework in the morning, house has gotta be kept clean and it clears my head of all the complexities of life at the moment. I got the train from Orpington to London Bridge. At London Bridge I made my usual way down the slope from the platform and as I got out of the station, I see the familiar faces and people in their jobs, people like the Shard security staff in their black overcoats, scarves and gloves, the beggars on the McDonalds steps and the Evening Standard guy giving the papers out etc, The volunteer Jehovah's witnesses giving out the magazines. All of these people would become part of my cancer journey, all involuntary witnesses to my treatment. They, of course, do not know that they are part of other peoples journeys too and not just mine, They have no idea that they are going to be mentioned in my book. Anyhow, I saw Dr P in clinic and as if I needed reminding, she told me that my disease was metastatic and my life expectancy was 18 months at the most but could be 12 months or less. She explained to Garreth and I that my cancer was no longer curable and my care was palliative care only. I cried and cried and hated this woman so much. However, I didn't feel sorry for myself, I did however feel so, so sorry for my Garreth. That poor boy had finally learned that his dad had been hand delivered a death sentence. She then dropped the bombshell that they are seriously considering adding another chemotherapy drug called CETUXIMAB to my list of chemo drugs by infusion but not for a couple of weeks yet. What a shock that was, and now I know that they really are trying to give me as much extra time to live as possible. I said my goodbye and we left the room and soon we were on our way to London Bridge Station. I was tired and as Gaz and I were on a packed train we were glad to get home safely and indoors in the warmth. Gaz and I talked about our day, it has to be talked about. It is good to discuss it between us, I was so glad that Gaz was with me to share this all. It is good that the extra chemo is being added to the mix. If it works for a lot of people then that's good enough for me. You never know, I might live longer than their 18 months estimated prediction of living. I now also know that my next chemo appointment day is January 20th and my next appointment to see Theresa etc is January 22nd. That too I hope is therefore a Wednesday. I think the 20th is a Monday. I didn't know, just as well Gaz was with me to tell me. Wednesday January 8th is over and tomorrow is a new day.

——— # # # ———

GOOD MORNING. It is Thursday January 9th 2014, this morning I feel one thing is certain which is that I have cancer but am now fighting it. This cancer of mine is not going to have an easy ride with me up against it. The changes and reactions have started however. One such change, which is very noticeable now, is I feel very, very cold all the time now and today, for the first time, I feel like I am going to be sick. This sickness feeling is totally new whereas the cold issue started last week. I have had only one heavy session of infused chemotherapy in Guys Hospital and then followed by 4 days of chemo going in 24/7. If you think about it, an awful lot of chemo has gone into my body which has never before in its life had any alien thing like chemo liquids going into it. It was only yesterday that I really only felt cold but this morning however is a whole new ball game completely. What a change in 24 hours. Another thing is that the lumps in my neck have not increased and unless I am imagining it, it seems that these lumps have even decreased in size a little. Maybe my mind is playing tricks or that I am hoping against all hope, but maybe the lumps have actually reduced. Am saying nothing to anyone at this stage, just in case it's a false alarm. Whether or not these good changes or bad changes are happening, I never ever in my life want to see this Dr P ever again. She is probably a lovely person but to me she is always the bearer of bloody bad news, but as long as she is part of the team, I cannot avoid her. I still absolutely adore my Consultant Theresa. She also happens to be the one that gives me good news or even not so bad news. I probably still need a consultant's true picture of things to get a proper idea of things. Either way I have f****** cancer and also now I am having the treatment that is the only way to treat it or deal with it. I know that it will never ever go away and I know that as I am now terminal and it is metastatic, it will win in the end and will kill me. I also know and remind myself every day that treatment is solely for one ultimate purpose and that is that the treatment is only buying me an extra bit of living time and if new things come on the market in the meantime, I may be lucky enough to be given something as a trial. I will make the most of today but to be honest it is getting very difficult to deal with this cancer thing. I always wondered how people coped with a death sentence. I wonder no more, now I am experiencing it in all its might. Tiredness and cold body temperatures alongside wanting to be sick are the current results of the day. Plenty more to follow, I'm sure. More tomorrow or later if I feel the need to put any incidents on paper, but if not then I will write tomorrow.

——— # # # ———

GOOD MORNING. Hi, it is Friday January 10th 2014 and it's my Wedding Anniversary. This day back in 1981, Joan and I were married so that makes it 33 years. Friday for most people is the end of the working week and therefore for many it is time to rest and recharge after a hard week at work. Then there is a person like me and while in this shitty position of carrying this fatal disease known to everyone as cancer, every day is now the same. I am sure by now you will have noticed from me a feeling of negativity. I expect this feeling will last quite a long time. I am angry, very angry. Why is it me? There are so many bad people in this world and nothing like this happens to them. I am not saying that I am a living saint but right now it seems so unfair or am I just being greedy. Right now, I would not want anyone of my family to be in my place. This is how I feel every day and night. As regards outside my family, then yes, I would swap right now. It is a horrible disease and I feel so messed up that I have it. Anyhow, today is just another day and the weekend is upon us. My sister called as usual earlier and we had a nice chat as we do every day now. Tomorrow is Saturday January 11th and as before, I am so cold and so very, very tired. As like yesterday, I am feeling sick but as yet have not got physically sick, yet! I will write tomorrow if I can.

——— # # # ———

Good Morning all. Yes it is Saturday January 11th 2014. I just want to explain to anyone reading this now that as time goes by with my condition from cancer or from treatment, there will be some days that I will not physically be able to write or that there will be no change in my condition to be interesting enough etc to write about. I will write of course whenever I can, but be prepared for blank days after which I will explain about on the next time of writing afterwards ... okay everyone, now I have explained that. I will now carry on but today is a quiet day. Please forgive me if my type of writing on particular days is a bit crap, but one reason for writing this is to show people how good or bad I feel as the days progress. Everybody is different and reacts differently but the results still are near enough the same in one form or another. I think I meet the team in 11 days from now. There is no scan in the meantime but on the day will be a visual check of the Lymph glands in the neck and throat externally as well as the possibility of a camera down the nostril into the back of the throat with just a spray numbing inside the nose. As you can imagine, it never numbs it enough so it is bloody horrible and brings tears to my eyes so the sooner it's over the better. It has to be done but not nice at all. Tomorrow is Sunday and if I feel okay in the morning it may be 10am Mass for me. Right now I know it's Winter but my body is freezing and the central heating in the house is up full.

——— # # # ———

GOOD MORNING. It is Sunday January 12th 2014 and as it is Sunday, a trip to Mass is on the cards this morning. My religion is important to me, not just now, but always has been. I pray now that my nearest and dearest Garreth will never have to go through the hell that I am going through now. I love that boy so much. He has gone through so much shit in his life but he is strong and coming through it. He lost his mum, my wife Joan, on November 16th 2008 and now he faces losing his dad. Anyhow, Mass was nice today, but so many people flocking around me again when they heard the news. Last Sunday I spoke to a few people and of course the fakes listening in, but word spreads of course. I need all the masses and prayers in the world now. It is certainly a very strange feeling thinking about my cancer. I am in my church where I go to as often as possible. This is the same church that my wife's funeral was in. I look back up behind me towards the top rows of seats near the altar and I'm thinking that whether this goes wrong sooner or later either way and if my consultant Theresa is right, I will be in a coffin in that same damn area near the altar and my funeral will be taking place. Eighteen months they reckon, so lets see if we all meet up back here sometime around June 23rd 2015, however, and there is always an "however"to put a spanner in the works. So, however, if I fight this like I intend to and try and kick cancer in the ass, there will be no funeral happening for me and those awaiting some thing in my will I'm afraid may have to accept the delay or even cancellation of my death. If that happens, all I can say is, sorry! I'm in a reflective mood today even a little sarcastic. I'd better get my ass in gear and contact Udens in Petts Wood. There is a guy there called Len who handled Joan's funeral, so I will be leaving instructions in the white envelope for him to be contacted at the time of my passing. Strange feeling that I have to think about death now. I get so many people saying to me that I shouldn't be talking or thinking like that, but, I'm the one with the bloody cancer, I'm the one going to die, so, it has to be done. Why wait until the end? I have to prepare now to ease the burden of my upcoming death sentence. Anyhow, I look at the watch and all this talking has to stop and I have to get home. Mass finished ages ago. I picked up the Parish Church Leaflet and left to go to my car and get home. At home, Sunday is such a long lazy day so no change there. The rest of the day went as smooth as possible. I feel tired, cold and feel sick. I have medication to take including anti-sickness liquid called Domperidone. Tomorrow is Monday January 13th so Cheerio for now. God Bless and take care ... xx

——— # # # ———

GOOD MORNING all, it is Monday January 13th 2014 and life goes on. Another feeling I get this morning is a very distinct wanting to be physically sick now, even more than before. I hate this nausea. I took my anti-sickness medicine Domperidone, disgusting stuff meant to stop me being sick but is in fact worse than puking up. No puking up yet but it's not far off. Puking up will happen and I have a list of all the other things expected to happen. Nausea is on the list and that is now out of the way and occurring on a daily basis. Let's get through the rest of today. No worry about my job. I am on long term sickness from my work and even though I would absolutely love to go back to work on my buses one day. Can you imagine the conversation. "There's that

Dave Cosgrave, he had terminal cancer and he beat it and came back to work". However, realistically I know that probably this will not happen but if it does, I will be in the history books for a different reason. So as for today, Cheerio and God Bless. See you tomorrow all. Yes tomorrow is Tuesday January 14th, another new day and another new feeling sick day with already feeling cold and very tired.

——— # # # ———

GOOD MORNING all. It is Tuesday January 14th 2014 and welcome to another new day and all that goes with it. I feel crap today. I felt sick during the night, hanging over the toilet bowl and feeling like I want to puke up but nothing came out. A completely new thing that I have noticed is a toilet issue. I apologise in advance now but it happened and will more than likely happen to some if not all cancer patients or cancer patients undergoing treatment of Chemotherapy. Okay here it is. I notice this morning a really awful putrid smell from my urine in the toilet bowl. It is a really awful smell and I make sure now that I flush the toilet now every time I pass urine. I do it anyway and have been doing it all my life but now I have to ensure that I do it now without fail. I also now notice that every time I pass urine it comes out so, so slow like a small trickle of water. A couple of days ago everything was okay but now suddenly things are going wrong. What is next to happen I ask myself, anything I suppose is possible. I have been given an absolutely huge list of things that could go wrong and a list of things that will for definite go wrong. There is no point for me to read off the list here now because quite simply some may or may not happen. There are various things on that list that are dependent on the amount of chemotherapy that I am having. My nausea at the moment is in the morning and if I take my anti-sickness in advance it will help to ease the number of times that I feel sick, however when the extra chemotherapy CETUXIMAB starts its infusion sessions, the amount of nausea and actual sickness will get worse. No amount of anti-sickness medication is guaranteed to have any effect on the nausea and the inevitable vomiting that lies ahead. Quite simply I do not know and that is probably for the best. I will deal with it if it happens or as it happens. Then the amount of vomiting will then create weakness in my body and that results then of further issue of "BUILD UP DRINKS" called "FORTISIP". Everything is dependent on future events, treatment and other medication. It can be crazy at times and I will need an awful lot of space for storage of all the medication and home treatments. Okay let me carry on but while I do not know what else is to happen, all I do know is the reason why! Simply, the reason is that I have cancer. Not a lot else is happening today. If there is then I will write it on here. My God it's cold, my whole body is cold even to touch on the outside. inside of course has been cold most of the time now for the past number of days and nights. Good Day to you all …

——— # # # ———

GOOD MORNING all. It is Wednesday January 15th 2014 and it is 3.20am. I have just had the most awful session of vomiting, violent vomiting and puking up of water etc. It ripped the stomach out of me. God Almighty it is still in the first month and I have so much to do and get through yet. I still have to face weeks and weeks and months and months of treatment and an extra introduction of that other chemotherapy called CETUXIMAB. There's going to be a lot more puking up like this morning just now and it will not be limited to the mornings, it's open season on vomiting for David now. My stomach is still sore and feels like it's been kicked, so I am going back to bed for rest and energy recovery. I will no doubt write later as it is very early in the day. Time is now 4.55am.

Well hello there again. Time is now 8.20am and both last night and this morning continue to be bad. Apart from the nausea, vomiting up whatever is in the stomach, feeling cold and shivery and absolutely stinking horrible smell from urine just passed. By the way that urine problem being smelly is simply maybe caused by the chemotherapy in my system reacting with whatever it comes in contact with and in this case the contents of my bladder namely urine. It will probably be for as long as I am having chemotherapy as a form of treatment. Anyway, this new problem to put up with is that many things are tasting like metal now or as dry and horrible like cardboard. So many things are now going that way that I am losing the taste for, so basically my taste buds for now have had it and that's what it's going to be like for a long way to go now. The taste buds are things that are gone for a long time with chemotherapy and radiotherapy. For now my problem is connected to Chemotherapy and those taste buds generally do not return for many weeks well after the end of chemotherapy infusion. The puking up has eased up a little for now. I am now taking loads of Domperidone anti-sickness. It's working for now so am going to take it well in advance to head off any chance of actually getting sick. The chemotherapy chemicals are hopefully working now or beginning to do some good and a lot will happen. I suppose in a way it's good to be getting sick as it shows that the chemotherapy is having an effect on me in there. Today I have an appointment in Guys Audiology at 3.30pm. I get a cab from home to Orpington Station and then the train to London Bridge. Then we have a short walk to Guys Hospital. Overall today is a bad day and to think about it is probably the first official bad day in my current shit situation. Bad day or not, I went to Guys Audiology and on getting there was told to go to the 10th floor for a blood test at 2.20pm. This was followed at 3.30pm with the actual Audiology appointment. I have absolutely no idea why I had an Audiology appointment but these wonderful people must know a reason for it. Bearing in mind the source of the cancer as it is head and neck is concentrated in an area at the base of the tongue at the back of the throat and a secondary cancer taking hold in my windpipe. If the chemo does not work, then all of this will be in vain. All the sickness, the thoughts running through my head, God please help me, my head for some reason is driving me mad more so this week than at any other time. The enormity of it all is suddenly poking its ugly head and I really do feel so much alone. I have Garreth in my life and nobody else. Oh yes, I have so many others but every one of them as far as I am concerned are Fakes. OK, Mary my sister, has gone out of her way for me and as said before still contacts me every day without fail and I have no reason to think that that will change at any time soon. Like Garreth, she is devastated. My Garreth is truly devastated but is slowly getting more able to bear up with the news. At the moment these are the only two people that I can genuinely say that they are in my life. Anyhow, my day in Guys is nearly over as basically all they wanted to see me for was because of the location of the cancer, my hearing and balance may be affected by any treatment. In a situation like mine and the cancer, after diagnosis all appropriate departments and experts in their field come on board and all departments kick in and work with each other at all stages during diagnosis, treatment and afterwards. It is all truly professional to see it all blending in and working together to make everything work successfully and properly. The NHS truly is a lovely gift that we all have and it must be treasured and looked after. Bless all the doctors, nurses and all consultants in the NHS. Time to get this packed train and get home. I also noticed this evening that a packed train is now getting difficult to cope with. I won't put up with it forever. For now it gets me home quickly or pretty quick. It's January, it's cold, so getting indoors is a priority and also tonight I have a district nurse coming round to flush out my PICC line. This is purely to check that there is no infection in the area and the actual treatment line was flushed through and that the line is actually clean and clear. Anyhow, I got home and so much for an early night, she came out late to do her cleaning and flushing of the line in my left arm. My early night went down the pan but lucky enough she didn't stay too long, just long enough to do cleaning correctly and write her report. I don't know what kept her writing but her writing took longer than her actual flushing and cleaning of my line for treatment. Apparently she is what is known as a "TWILIGHT NURSE". My twilight nurse left in her twilight transport into the twilight night. Gaz and I had a catch up of the day's events. Then it was bedtime and whatever I was facing during the night. As my treatment progresses, anything can happen now either day or night. Meanwhile, Goodnight all.

——— # # # ———

GOOD MORNING all. It is Thursday January 16th 2014 and surprise, surprise, no puking up last night or this morning yet. I slept well and now, before I forget it, my next big event is on Wednesday 22nd January 2014. That day I see my consultant Theresa Guerrero-Urbano and get a treatment progress report. My taste buds are rapidly going now. Most things taste now like paper or metallic. The list of changes to my body is absolutely endless so as it happens I will let you know here. I have no doubt that very soon they will all show or begin to show themselves to me in one form or another. Right now it's a waiting game. As to what happens next is anybody's guess. Cold and tired now, it's a short report today so Cheerio to you all.

——— # # # ———

Good Day to you all. It's Friday January 17th 2014. So I should say, Good morning all and like I said before the end of the week for many working people where they re charge their body batteries all weekend and back to work on Monday morning. In my case however, like many cancer patients, life carries on. My case is also different now because my body is taking a pounding 24/7. Again, no getting sick last night, but as the chemo is now going around in my bloodstream and is reaching every nook and cranny in my body. I would love to know if anything good is happening inside my body right now. On Wednesday 22nd I should have an idea, I could be wrong but the lumps in my neck do actually seem not to have grown in size, in fact they actually seem to be shrinking. Can this really be happening after such a short time on chemotherapy. It could be one of my false hopes. There is nothing worse than building hopes up and then have those hopes come crashing down to earth with reality. Good day and goodnight all. I am chilled to the bone...

——— # # # ———

Good day to everyone. It is Saturday January 18th 2014. Sorry. nothing out of the ordinary today. Let's see what tomorrow brings. I am taking it easy today and bring on tomorrow Sunday.

——— # # # ———

GOOD MORNING ALL. It's Sunday January 19th 2014 and as it's Sunday, that means Mass Day. My God it has come around so quickly. Everybody so concerned but as we have already seen many times, hiding in my religion are the fakes. They pretend to care and as far as they are concerned it's all about spreading gossip and false stories. They also add tails to their stories and spread it as soon as it is what they want it to be. As soon as the actual truth emerges, they hide and are nowhere to be seen. One place you will never find them is the confession box. Still, I do pray a lot, I need my religion and even more now. I actually believe that my God will help me. If he wants me to live or just live longer, he will sort it out. If he wants me to die and go to him, then I am ready. Let's see ... Tomorrow is Monday January 20th ... Good night all. I am on borrowed time.

——— # # # ———

Good Morning everyone, it is Monday January 20th 2014. Where do I begin. Getting anxious now with 2 days to go before I meet my Consultant Theresa for the first time since beginning treatment. I realise that there has been no scan and there won't be for some time yet but I still want to see the team that are trying to keep me alive. At the last meeting of the team back on January 8th. It was just awful being told that my disease is no longer curable. Therefore I am on borrowed time and when you think about it, I have borrowed it from that clever person or persons that created my batch of overall chemotherapy. However, this borrowed time is running out. As for today, Monday 20th is a normal Monday. All over the world people are being born and people are dying. People are getting good news and bad news. The world population is always changing by the second or millisecond. As for today in my case, nothing special. I suppose in a way I have a lot to be thankful for. My son Garreth is in a brilliant job with fantastic prospects. Okay, I have Cancer but even though I have a death sentence hanging over me. I am fighting to live and I will continue to fight and fight and fight unless the cold and tiredness gets me first. Good Day and Good Night to you all.

——— # # # ———

Good Morning all. It's early hours of Tuesday January 21st 2014 and I am looking out my window on to my empty street, my empty lonely street and most people sleeping. I then think how many of my neighbours are lying there awake and thinking about their lives and their problems. Everyone has problems in life. It's quiet outside and I am awake because I have just been vomiting a lot. This morning I have something new, yes, a rash on my face. This rash is new and is on the list. It's weird seeing me ticking off the boxes that these people tell me what will happen. As I look on to the street again, I just spotted the milkman in his van delivering. It's 4.15am. I must get back to bed and get some more sleep. I hope no more sick this morning so will write later when I wake up again.

Well good morning again. After last night and the puking episode, I did manage to get some sleep. It's cold outside today but that's what you get in

January. It may be cold and I may be a little tired but many people will not be alive in a few minutes time and that simply is life. I am no longer scared of dying. I watched my late wife Joan pass away and it was so peaceful. I want to go like that when it is my time to go. It may seem strange talking about death but the experts have told me that the inevitable is going to happen for me eventually so as well as treatment, I also have to prepare myself for it and accept my fate. So good all. Tomorrow I meet Theresa and the team responsible for planning, preparing and issuing the various chemotherapy chemicals and infusing them into me. Until then, let's get some well earned sleep. Goodnight to each and every one of you.. xx

——— # # # ———

Hi all... It is Wednesday January 22nd 2014 and today is one hell of a big day. I certainly do not want to meet Dr P as she only delivers bad news to me. I want Dr Theresa Guerrero-Urbano. Theresa is a lady that I have developed a trust of. She means well and does well. Today I took the usual method of transport. The cab from home to the station. In the cab the conversation led to my reason for travelling and my cancer. The driver too had family with cancer. Nowadays everybody has been visited by cancer. It affects so many people nowadays. At the station I gave him the £5 fare plus the tip. At Orpington station, I met Peter and Roxy, some platform staff who I would get to know pretty well eventually as my treatment progressed in Guys Hospital in London. I then got the fast train from platform 2 to London Bridge. At London Bridge I met my son Gaz who took time off work. Gaz would from now on be with me in on all consultant appointments. I had some spare time so I popped into MacDonalds for a large fries and a vanilla shake. I can't remember what Gaz had. It was a quick visit and we made our way to Guys Hospital nearby. We were a little early arriving at Guys for our 3.20pm appointment in Oncology Outpatients and checked in. I was weighed and had a blood test. Before I go any further, let me explain something to you. I had a massive life threatening heart attack in 2007. At the time I was over 24 stone (146 kilos) in weight. That was May 13th 2007, I never forget it. I went on a waiting list for gastric band surgery. My wife Joan saved me that night by calling an ambulance as soon as I got the first small pain. Sadly we lost Joan on November 16th 2008. I had my Bariatric surgery on May 1st 2009. As a result my weight is today 82 kilos, a loss of 64 kilos. The band now has maximum restriction. I can only eat a little, but all the tiny amount is disgusting as it tastes like paper or metal. Great eh! We waited and waited. Eventually Theresa's clinic was running about an hour late. I noticed that some clinics were running on time or maybe 15 to 20 minutes late. Theresa's was running late as was another clinic and the reason is the same for both. Theresa was running late because of her personality. She is the type of person that does not rush her patients. She takes time with every person especially those that have a terminal diagnosis. Because of this human touch, she runs late. This would be the case therefore in most of her clinics as I would later find out. Eventually I was called and Gaz and I went into the Consultation room. Garreth's girlfriend at the time was with us too. Theresa told me that I had to get used to realizing that any chemotherapy treatment was just for only improving my survival and as a result my quality of life. Quality of life was the most important and does not necessarily go hand-in-hand with getting borrowed time. Getting extra time to live, sometimes does not always lead to quality of life. I told her that I coped well so far with the first bout of Chemotherapy but tiredness was an issue and I felt cold and very cold quite often over the first few weeks even though the chemo only was treatment for one week even if it was intense. I told her that to be honest it was a struggle at times. Theresa then told me that I had seen nothing yet as regards reaction to chemotherapy. She said that coming up would be reactions that would result in me at times wishing that I hated life and that the most horrendous time was on its way. She told me to prepare for PERIPHERAL NEUROPATHY, a numbness or lack of feeling and sometimes tingling or pins and needles in the nerve endings of fingers, toes or feet. Sometimes all at the same time and there is a lot more to come. Today for example is something new, dry sore eyes. My God, these changes to my body are all suddenly happening to me. Theresa prescribed HYPROMELLOSE eye drops and she then told me that in the coming weeks things will gradually worsen over time. Then she gave me the bombshell, which I had been half expecting but it was still a shock. It was that in five days from today on January 27th a further drug called CETUXIMAB would be introduced. I asked why and she said that on an external examination of my neck, there was a slightly noticeable reduction in the external size in the lymph nodes (lumps) on my neck. In other words after a couple of weeks I have had a very good partial response to the chemotherapy treatment by CISPLATIN and 5FU that I've already had. The lumps have reduced on the left side of my neck mainly, however, the remaining worry in my neck is palpable lymph node 2cms in size in a post auricular level 5 region. I have absolutely no idea what she means by that, but I do know that basically response is good to treatment, some lumps reduced but some not and the secondary cancer is probably still in the windpipe. Because there is no scan, there is no idea how it is behaving. Only a Pet Scan will give a proper result. My blood count is satisfactory for going ahead with the extra CETUXIMAB Chemotherapy on the 27th January. This now also means that I will be having intense Chemotherapy every week in Guys Cancer Day Unit. Basically now it means also that they will do a PET Scan after 3 cycles to assess my overall response. In laymans terms the future now will be hell on earth as the Chemotherapy levels build up in my body attacking this bloody cancer. My cancer is aggressive and is doing its level best to kill me.

The chemo is now going to be hitting me back on 3 sides in my attempt to fight back and guess what, I am in the middle of it all getting hit by cancer and hit by chemotherapy. One of them will win, no middle ground. My treatment therefore will be in Guys and is easy to work out... WEEK 1. Cisplatin, 5FU, Cetuximab and 5FU PUMP (at home for a further 5 days over 24/7 and then disconnection by district nurse and flushing). WEEK 2... 5FU and Cetuximab infusion. WEEK 3... Cetuximab infusion. That then is the end of one cycle of 3 weeks. My treatment is over a period of 6 cycles (18 weeks) ... In 3 cycles (9 weeks) from now there will therefore be a PET Scan. Then and only then will we know if the treatment will be working or not. I will see Theresa at the end of every cycle. At the rate that I am now suddenly getting sick and the horrible changes happening within my body, I expect to be far, far worse while the chemo which will now be 3 drugs takes hold of my body. I now know that suddenly things are getting far, far worse for me. I like Theresa and even though Gaz was with me, I suddenly burst into tears. Weeks of pressure was building up inside of me and now I was going to emotionally let rip. I cried and cried and cried. Just think only a week ago, I guessed my reaction was getting strange but now inside me I was cracking up. For the first time ever I hated all healthy people around me. I detested healthy people. I was going to have to go through absolute hell to have any chance whatsoever. As I said before and I apologise if I repeated the following but coming up will be a nasty overall reaction to me and anybody who gets close to me. I will have to try to balance out my trips to see Milena in Razgrad, Bulgaria and have my treatment. Obviously treatment will take priority but I can also try to do the two. I am a fighter so I will fight to do both. For the record, my exact cancer locations etc are as follows ... T2 N3 M1(SCC) OROPHARYNX (LEFT BASE OF TONGUE BASE) METASTATIC DISEASE TO THE MEDIASTINAL NODES CONFIRMED BY EBUS AND FNA.

My care is Palliative over 6 cycles. 6 cycles is 18 weeks. So eighteen weeks of intense chemotherapy. My prescriptions are now free and numerous in types of Medication. Eventually my crying eased. I left Theresa's room a broken man. She gave me helpful news but only a scan will tell the true story. There are going to be so many tearful nights coming up now and I again cannot help notice that suddenly it is all happening. The train home was a packed one. I looked around me. How many of these passengers all around me had cancer hidden amongst them. My eyes were already getting sore and hurting. Without a mirror I cannot tell but I can only also assume that they are reddening up too. I need to get home. When I think back to today, it was good to hear from Theresa even though it was a comment based on a visual check, that my neck lumps may be easing in size etc. However, deep inside in me this horrible disease in the beastly form called Cancer. It is doing its silent, dark and dirty work. I just want to lock myself away now and wake up tomorrow to realize it is all a bad dream, but it's not a dream and this is my only opportunity to put every gruesome detail down here. Many of you reading this may be doing so for the first time to understand how to get to grips in the form of a daily blog of what it is like to live with and deal with Cancer. It is also about getting to grips with a Cancer sufferer's getting used to the fact that this Cancer is going to kill me. Cancer is probably one of the most awful six letter words in the English language. I sometimes think who on earth was the first person to get Cancer and where in their body did they have it. I wonder how did they deal with the pain and the mental torture of it all. their families, loved ones, how did the various people affected by it actually deal with it.

So many of you will be reading this, not as a long-term patient, but possibly as a carer, a relative or friend or in the horrible scary position of just been tested and awaiting a diagnosis but deep down you know that you have it but must still await that visit to the consultant where you are advised to bring someone with you. Let me tell you that if it is the case where you are advised to bring someone with you, please do not tear yourself apart because of this advice. Bring someone with you is also because there may be nothing in your scan results but believe you me, you will need a hand to grip for both types of results. You may have yourself all worked up and then nothing and your mind goes blank. There and then is where you will need someone to lean on, good or bad. Some of you reading this may be an Oncologist getting a perspective on the disease. If you are a relative or carer, you may be trying to understand what it does to the sufferer. You may be a scientist or a person about to release a cancer drug on to the market or maybe you cannot decide what to charge for it and you are looking for what it actually is to be a sufferer and your drug can make a difference to life getting hope in a drug. Maybe you are a hospital receptionist and you have no idea what a cancer sufferer or their family goes through on a daily or hourly basis. Let me ask you one question. Do you have a hard exterior where nothing flinches you or is it a weak one where the mere mention of the word puts the fear of hell into you. Everyone is different but my pain is two fold, physical pain and personal pain realising that I am going to die from this beast inside me. The physical pain will get worse as the treatment progresses with its numerous side effects and as the Cancer takes hold, that pain too. I can promise you one thing, the side effects on me now, after only a few weeks, are already simply awful and are going to be even more horrible on a daily basis. Three weeks ago I was in the very early stages of chemotherapy. Now it's 3 drugs in and it's bed sore eyes, vomiting, freezing cold body, tiredness, confusion, no taste buds and crying at random without any warning or expectation, yes me born in 1957 as I write, a grown man crying and no special reason why I cry. Already it's hell on earth, nobody has any idea what I am going through right now. Unless you have cancer or have had it, then you just do not bloody know. When you walk in my shoes, only then do you know. Before I close for the day, very soon the weight loss will begin to happen, followed by the hair loss. The hair loss will probably as I said not really affect me as I am as bald as "THE KING BALDY OF ALL THE BALDIES IN BALDYVILLE" now that's what you call bald. I always said that grass doesn't grow on a busy street. But for now, Goodnight all and may your God get you through the night and may the same God wake you up tomorrow morning. I may say goodnight but it's only goodnight from writing. I will probably watch some TV to take my mind off of everything. Talk tomorrow all... xx

——— # # # ———

Hello all, it's THURSDAY JANUARY 23rd 2014 and I am blubbering here, a grown man crying my eyes out and just thinking. I think when is it going to end and then I realise that it's only just begun. Long road ahead and I have no idea if I can get through it all. I feel so alone, got to get MacMillan on board soon. Now to get some more sleep. This crying is random and no warning at all of it happening. All new stuff to me and I wish I knew what was next in these surprises. Back to bed for me now.

Morning all, still Thursday January 23rd and it's 10am. I just had a phone call from GUYS ONCOLOGY. The introduction of the new Chemotherapy drug CETUXIMAB is now not going ahead as planned for tomorrow 24th. It has been delayed because they could not get it ready on time. The results of my urea and electrolytes were not back in time for their readings to be studied in order for my dose of CETUXIMAB to be suitably prepared. However, it is going ahead on next Monday 27th January 2014. As I already said my prescriptions are now free, so I need to live as long as possible to get maximum from it all. Nothing else to add today apart from my own other personal thoughts. Every day I ask myself one question ... WHY ME? Only my God above knows and as good as he is, I'd rather not meet him yet... OK. Goodnight all.. xx

——— # # # ———

GOOD MORNING EVERYONE. It is Friday January 24th 2014. I had a reasonable night. Body feels cold all the time. Had a call from Garreth earlier. I don't know how he settles his mind at his work with my problems hitting him. He's a strong boy, I love him to bits. I am very, very proud of him and what he has achieved, University, Graduation and Work. My employers are still paying me full sick pay. I am growing more and more tired now and some days what I do is exactly what I am doing today. After getting up and taking my heart medication, I am after having a shower and back in my dressing gown and lying on the bed followed by me then even getting back under the covers of that same bed. Again today another call. All treatment including the new CETUXIMAB will now be going ahead on Monday 27th at 10.30am and with the other drugs again on Tuesday 28th at 10.30am ... Sorry, I am wiped out and will write tomorrow.

——— # # # ———

Hi all ... it's SATURDAY JANUARY 25th 2014. I am so cold and extremely tired and cold. My heating is up full and earlier I cried and vomited a little. I am sorry but will. try again tomorrow. This is truly awful but I have to go.

——— # # # ———

Good day to everyone. It's Sunday January 26th 2014 and today is a repeat of yesterday. Plenty of Sleep, vomiting, thinking and crying. This crying makes me look like a depression fuelled human being. No day goes by without feeling lonely, lost vomiting and crying. My God I was told about this but I am not prepared for any of this. Just look at it all weekend lost because of vomiting, thinking, cold and crying. My life is getting unbearable now. What an exciting life I lead. Can you imagine if all your life consisted of those basic things that I have been doing and I still await the surprises linked to the disease and the remaining treatment. My life is now effectively on hold. Work has stopped but I may go back if I am well enough after treatment. Realistically because my disease is terminal, I doubt if it is going to happen. My employers will soon start pushing for full termination of my employment. I am already too tired to fight so I think the inevitable is going to happen. They know not to pester me too much and of course I have my consultant and MacMillan on my side. Anyhow tomorrow is Monday 27th and my 2nd cycle of Chemo is now on the day after at 10.30am but Cetuximab is tomorrow, also at 10.30am. In a way it will certainly be different as my journey continues. My diaries are all up to date and my diary entries and updates are all here, nothing omitted. Goodnight all. Sleep well and I may be talking to you later depending on my Domperidone anti-sickness not to be confused with a similar sounding named Champagne. Great isn't it. One is a free prescription and the other I cannot afford. Goodnight xx

——— # # # ———

Morning. Monday January 27th 2014 and it was too good to be true. Yes the usual vomiting but surprise surprise, something very new. I have a slight sight of rash on the left side of my face which has to be a reaction to all that chemo some time ago. Nothing surprises me now and gotta get back to bed. It's 5am, too bloody early so talk or write later.

Hi there, 5am was dark, it's now 8am and a more reasonable time of the day to write. I am quite surprised that this rash or redness is showing. Better keep an eye on it in case it gets worse. While all this is happening, I have a daily lot of medication to take. Some of it is for a heart attack in 2007 and some as part of my cancer treatment. As you know the chemo is now making me sick quite a lot now. The anti-sickness medication tastes disgusting. There is no other taste like it. Even sometimes the anti-sickness medication makes me want to heave and puke up. That sounds a bit Irish but it's true, it does. Then there are the injections where I inject myself into the wall of my belly alternate sides on alternate days for blood thinning. Then there are the injections into my upper thigh which are for white cell boosting purposes. The chemo has reduced or destroyed the white cells and these injections counteract this happening or ,at the very least, help to boost the white cells. I also take paracetamol soluble and vitamin pills. I rattle when I walk. As before, I have to make the most of today. I just need to get to Guys as quickly as possible and have my Cetuximab infusion. Then, when that's over, get my appointment card and get home as fast as possible. Tomorrow I am facing all 3 drugs Chemotherapy infusion including, again, the new Cetuximab. I got back home after 3pm. I am tired and feeling very sleepy. Probably a very early night for me as nothing else to do. Talk tomorrow. Goodnight all.

——— # # # ———

GOOD MORNING ALL. It is Tuesday January 28th 2014. It is a very important day for me and my Oncology team in Guys. I am at Guys later for the second introduction of CETUXIMAB, on top of my other chemo drugs. It is now 8.30am so gotta get my ass in gear and get up to London and Guys Hospital. Cab is booked for 9.15am for a train around 9.30am or so. I have no idea what to expect with this new chemo drug introduction. I do know that it is by the usual method of infusion into my arm via my PICC Line. We are only 26 days in and look what 5 or 6 days of chemo has already done to me. I have such a long way to go yet and at this stage, as you know, I feel like absolute shit. My whole life is on hold and when it comes to dating, I have to be honest and straight with anyone I do meet. I don't think it's fair on any person I would meet, not to tell them that I have cancer. Cancer is such a dealbreaker. If I met anybody then it's a case of, are they taking a chance on me, or are they the type to use my sickness to get what they can. At the moment I am in a relationship with Milena at Razgrad in Bulgaria. Soon I will be given a chemo break and go and see her. For all I know she may be seeing someone else. What can I do but keep my side of the deal and stay loyal? I am getting too sick to keep two women going so I will stick to the one, even though it is a long distance relationship. As for my cancer and Milena, I do not know. So many people are telling me to be careful but as I said, I will be careful. I hope she is with me for who I am. Let's see what happens here then. In the long run, I cannot see it last a long time. I will not be moving there. My home is here and I will never, ever leave the side of my son Gaz. He is my world. That is a promise to Garreth. I (his dad) will never leave his side. As for today, now I know my way.

As I got to the front of Guys Hospital, those two stupid revolving doors, and it's always the pricks on mobiles not concentrating on the matter in hand are the pricks that rush the doors and always mess it up. The door jams up and everything stops. The ones that cause it then look up from their phones and then look around to try to pass the blame. ASSHOLES! After it frees itself, I make my way past the coffee area. I went straight for the correct lift to get me to the 10th floor and the Cancer Day Unit. Anybody who is in this lift and gets off at this floor is linked, without doubt, to cancer. On this 10th floor you are either staff, visitor, patient escort, patient, consultant or nurses. I made my way to the desk now getting to know the girls and the one bloke Richard. Today, Evelyn is on the front desk with Richard. Heena is in the office making the appointments to all the little blue books and to my little blue appointment book. I get my wristband with all my details. Weird getting a wristband with info on it including my date of birth, my full name. It's like on holiday and getting all inclusive chemotherapy and in a way that's exactly what it is. I take my place in the waiting area. Sometimes they take patients into a side room for weight and blood testing. As the chemo treatment progresses, obviously the insides are changing all the time and blood levels change as it takes hold. Eventually, it may get to the point where I will be like a pin cushion by having blood tests every single week. Anyhow, I am still waiting and it's near 11am well past my 10.30am appointment time. Nearby is another waiting area on this 10th floor area in the Cancer Day Unit. This other area has soft armchairs, TV, tea, coffee, soft drinks, fresh fruit and two (2) wireless internet posts. I am in the other area near the front desk and Lucy, one of the cancer nurses calls, my name. It is 11.40am. This is it, Day one of the big 3, CISPLATIN, 5FU and CETUXIMAB. The introduction of Cetuximab was planned by Theresa my consultant. Now it's time for it's 2nd big introduction by infusion. I hope it goes ok being so soon after yesterday's introduction. Lucy is Irish as are so many of the nurses in the NHS. In this cancer unit there also are so many Irish nurses. I cannot remember the exact cubicle location but I was shown to my cubicle where, as before, there are 4 seated areas with loungers and infusion trolleys. Earlier I had a quick blood test when I came in first. I now realise the delay was because they had to wait for my blood test results to come back so that they had the all clear to go ahead with my 3 chemo drugs. It was going to be a long day and around 1.30pm Garreth was due down from work after taking his lunch break to sit with me. However, that was later on but for now my infusion was going ahead. Around me I noticed the few patients receiving chemo but looking like jockeys with their helmets. As I said these helmets are headgear with cold water running through them near the scalp as it helps patients that have treatment to not lose their hair. I was soon being prepared for my infusion by having the PICC Line in my arm being flushed through. Various packs of fluid was loaded up and connected up to me. I love the Piriton which makes me sleepy. Love it all here now, wrapped up in a blanket, feet up and nodding off. Eventually the chemo is connected up. I look around and most here seem asleep or eyes close being rested, even those with visitors or carers with them. Having chemo just wears a body down. It just knocks the absolute shit out of everyone. It destroys you, wipes you out and as the treatment progresses, the person having the chemotherapy just sleeps and sleeps and sleeps. Having chemo forces you to cancel ordinary living. You just exist in your own world and nobody understands that unless they have been through it. If they say "I understand", that's absolute bo***x. They simply are being apologetic, they haven't a f****** clue.

Anyhow back to today's treatment, my all inclusive wristband entitles me to have something from the snacks trolley as it comes around, but depending on pot luck to which ever side she starts her trolley trip, when she gets to you there may only be a few bits remaining to eat. Tea and coffee never runs out. Over the course of the next few hours my chemo infusion carried on via my PICC Line which uses the blood flow and the pumping of my heart, to basically suck in the liquid chemo and pump it around the blood system and eventually into every part of the body where blood goes, in effect, everywhere. So even the chemo goes with the flow. All cells die at the hands of the chemo but healthy and reasonably healthy ones eventually recover but the bad cells are killed off and never recover, hence the reason why it takes such a long time to recover from chemotherapy.

Sorry if I keep drifting away from writing about my actual treatment. I can tell you one thing, once the fluid of any kind starts going into the body and in this case mine, I was constantly going to the loo. I never stopped passing urine and of course what goes in, must come out and in my case it felt like gallons of urine. It was unbelievable the amount of it. Garreth came to sit beside me and it was great to have him with me. I don't know if he has noticed any changes in me from the Chemotherapy. I know one thing. I can see small gradual changes now on a daily basis. Sometimes changes are by the hour. Garreth, or as everyone calls him Gaz, had to leave and return to work but it was great to see him and I was awake while he came to be with me. It's now getting late in the day but I cannot see myself leave here until 5.30 or 6.00pm. Anyhow the chemo drugs are progressing and the last one, the new one called CETUXIMAB is about to be put into me. This CETUXIMAB is supposed to be the revolutionary drug in my case to give me extended life, or in effect allowing me to buy a little extra time to live. As my infusion machine is set up with the rate of infusion entered into it, I was drifting off to sleep again. Nothing wrong with that. I will sleep while this chemo is getting pumped into me. No going back now. If Theresa says it is going do me good, then and up to now she has done nothing for me to doubt her judgement, so I am happy that her judgement controls and decides this. As far as I am concerned, Theresa can do no wrong. She is a very clever woman and she has said she will do as much as possible to allow me to live longer than expected following my diagnosis. The prognosis of 18 months to live continues but can you imagine if I get the miracle gift of extra time living now, how good is that eh! I know that I have drawn the short straw and I know that death is going to come to me earlier than expected.

Anyhow, I slept and woke up to a nurse disconnecting me from my CETUXIMAB treatment bag of liquid tricks. This magic clear liquid is now in me and it is 5.40pm. The nurse still has to flush the line out and "have a chat". This time I knew what the chat was. It was about keeping rested and keeping the PICC Line clean and protected. She also explained that because it was a full day of treatment of 3 separate chemo drugs and now followed by having my chemo pump connected up to me, my body would be hit by unprecedented unknown extreme crippling tiredness, nothing like I have previously known. I was advised that if travelling home by train, to get on it and get home within a few hours before exhaustion would hit me. Within 24 hours I would definitely know about it.

Eventually after all the flushing was done and the pump full of 5FU was connected up. I made my plans to leave. I went to get my jacket and got such a shock after I fell back in my chair lounger. I was wiped out but I knew that I had to get to that loo or else wet myself. Falling back into the chair frightened me. I was wiped out beyond understanding and describing what has come over me in the space of a couple of hours, ok not a couple of hours but maybe 9 or 10 or so. I cannot believe or understand the destruction of my energy levels. I was alone and I burst out crying, alone, helpless and feeling like I was the loneliest man on earth. I cried for many reasons but mainly because I was alone and the cancer was in charge. It was then that I felt that the cancer and the chemo were working side by side together against me and also in a way fighting each other to gain the upper hand as to which one was in control of me. I was in the middle of the two and I didn't matter. I was now also, as a result, becoming irritable. All my life I was never really irritable, never, never, never. Now these two both the drugs and the chemo had done it to me. I was now trapped in a life that was now on hold and I had no idea how long that hold would last. So now to put it all together, alone, the weakling, trapped, tired, sick and now on hold going nowhere for the immediate future. My life now was a most awful place to be in. I felt unloved and ugly and I felt that everyone in this Cancer Day Unit was looking at me and after all that has just happened, maybe they were. Suddenly, a nurse in charge who I would later get to know as Aoife, an Irish nurse, came to my side gave me a hug, held my hand and suddenly made me good again. A nurse, who like all nurses, was just there and "nursed"me. That is all it took and I felt human and loved and cared for all over again. We talked with low voices and what a difference Aoife made. Aoife didn't need to have any wonderful medication with her. All she had was her caring voice and a simple human touch. It worked and I felt a little better again. Aoife was my angel. Her actions had dispelled any negative feelings that I had. As she spoke to me my tears flowed too. Her words and actions and simple just listening to me was enough to take the torment and pain away. Maybe the same gesture from any human being would have been enough to achieve the same result. A simple random act of kindness was all it took. Aoife left to do what she was earlier doing and I again attempted to try to leave to go home. This time it worked and I put on my jacket and left the Unit. I have no doubt that it would be repeated several times over again and while this is only a few weeks into my treatment, my God, just look at how things have changed for me in such a short space of time. I would soon learn and it's already showing in the early stages of my cancer journey that just the basic human contact is the greatest gift next in importance to actual state of health.

After the intervention of Aoife, I was just strong enough to make my way home. Under my clothing I could feel the bulky package that I was now wearing and my God it was bulky and awkward and a little heavy as it was draped across my chest from top left shoulder down to right waist. Aoife was busy so I just called her name and simply said "thank you and goodbye". I spotted Lucy who, like Aoife, was still working having been there since around 8am that morning. It was after 7pm, I collected my blue appointment card booklet and noticed that I was due back here for more chemo next Monday February 3rd 2014. Anything was now likely to happen between now and then. I made my way to the lift. On reaching the ground floor, I made my slow tedious walk to London Bridge Station. I texted Gaz and told him that I was near the station and that I just wanted to sleep as soon as I got home. I was lucky as the rush hour was easing off. I got a fast train to Orpington and then a taxi home. I felt a little strange on the train with my pump etc hidden under my clothes, just shows that anybody really can hide anything under their clothes well concealed amongst a lot of people even though the crowds were easing. Like I said, anything can be hidden. As soon as I got in I had a quick very sweet tasting cup of tea. I secured the house, turned up the heating, took my medication and went to bed. I was so exhausted, I really did not care when I woke up, I just wanted sleep. I texted Gaz to say I was home safe indoors and also to my sister Mary a similar message. I had no energy to talk to anyone. I assume that sleep came quickly because the last thing I noticed was my clock at 8.30pm. I awoke again quickly at about 11pm vomiting and feeling lost. I was lucky to have tissues beside me as I vomited. It was mainly clear liquid but it hurt my stomach while I was vomiting. I hadn't eaten a lot because of this metallic taste in my mouth. As I was alone, I hated my situation but nothing I could do about it. I fell back to sleep again and did not wake till near 10am this morning.

——— # # # ———

YES… This morning is Wednesday January 29th 2014. I just could only lay in bed and thought, My God, yesterday was such an exhausting day. So much happened. Everything happened and right now I can do nothing but lie here for now. If this is what is going to happen from here on, how the hell can I get through it all and on my own. Okay I got Gaz with me and I am so lucky to have him but there is no one but Gaz to help me so Bless him for that. He's such a great person to have as a son. Thank you Gaz, looks like it's just the two of us. It's going to be a hell of a battle with no guarantee of a successful outcome. They said it would happen within 24 hours. Well it has, well and truly. Today is a day of rest and updating my diary and whatever is in that diary will definitely end up on here. More rest is needed today. My God, what a change since last week. I am absolutely wiped out. Yes my chemo pump is showing a little sign of getting smaller in the balloon. I just realised, too, that this is my second pump as well so things are now really getting serious, anyhow all is well and I don't mean to cut things short. So. Sorry! I will write here again as soon as I can.

——— # # # ———

THURSDAY JANUARY 30TH 2014. NO COMMENT TODAY, just to say that the chemotherapy pump is really getting noticeably smaller today, bye xx

——— # # # ———

Good Morning, FRIDAY. January 31st 2014. Hi all. It is just after 8am. I have a taxi on the way at 9.15 to catch a train after 9.30 for a 10.15am appointment in Guys with a psyschotherapist called M S. What do I know? I have never met her or even heard about her. I don't even know what to do, but someone has said that I have to see her. I imagine it is to see how I am coping or dealing with the idea that in effect my diagnosis is a death sentence and at every scan result in future that death sentence is affirmed if the results are bad and delayed if results are good. Now you may notice that I say delayed rather than cancelled. When it comes to prognosis, cancelling is not used. Cancelling means I am cured and the cancer is gone. In my case my cancer is metastatic and therefore is eventually going to kill me. So M. S. wants to see me. I went to her Department of Psychotherapy and made myself known to her. I was already very tired from just a simple journey by train to London Bridge Station followed by a walk to the hospital. Anyhow, I am here now and what's up next? Oh dear, what a cock up, bloody hilarious. She doesn't ever want to see me again. A tall woman came out to the waiting room and like a missile scanning for its target, she scanned the room. There was probably about 8 or 9 in the room including me. We all looked up of course, like anxious chickens looking for food. Picture the scene, this woman who at this stage more of us knew who she was but she didn't have a clue who she was looking for. Not one of us were in any mood to suggest anything to her. Wearing a yellow top, black skirt and knee high boots like Dick Whittington in Puss in Boots, she stopped scanning and went about turn and then started ticking off a name on the clipboard at the same time as announcing "David Cosgrave, is there a Mr Cosgrave here?" I knew immediately that this was not going to have a happy ending, but whatever the ending was going to be, I thought, you know what, I am already in shit street having cancer and the chances were that this dominatrix of a woman was the psychotherapist herself and that she was going to see me and her cold bossy manner may be lovely to those that mattered to her in life but to me it looked like that there was more life in a wet fart on a cold damp Friday afternoon. I followed her to the door of a small room and she held it open and said the magic words "After you Mr Cosgrave, please take a seat". I duly obliged and my first unintentional action set the scene and ruined her day while making mine. It was enough to destroy things where she soon lost control of the whole matter.

I did was sit in a chair, a simple act for an average human being to achieve. There were two chairs in that room and yes, you may or may not have guessed, but I sat in the wrong bloody chair. This was not going to go well. I remained seated in my selected chair while this woman sat opposite me. As we sat opposite each other we of course looked at each other she suddenly said to me "Hello Mr Cosgrave, my name is M S and thank you for coming to see me today". Yes, that was her, the same name on my appointment letter. She was a medical professional in the system to see how I was coping. She was probably a lovely person and welcomed me and asked me if anything was troubling me. I told her that I was okay and everything was okay as regards me dealing with my cancer. This woman is part of a fantastic team or regime that automatically kicks in when a person is told devastating news, like me being told that I had terminal cancer. Our NHS is absolutely brilliant, so therefore this woman is also probably brilliant in her job but I soon knew that it wasn't for me. She told me that she assumed that my diagnosis was so awful, did I have any thoughts of ending my life by my own hand in other words, have I considered suicide in any form. I did not want to hear this because quite simply, I am not that type of person.

From Day 1 when told of my terminal cancer stage 4 now, I decided to fight to live. I had the cancer and how or why I got it didn't matter. It wasn't going to change the eventual outcome and I just want to take the treatment offered. So many people are not offered treatment because things are gone too far to have any hope. I wanted every possible hope available to extend my life. So no, suicide or assisted death is not for me. Anyhow the lady done something that made me very uneasy and I realised, through no fault of anyone, that this meeting was going down the pan. Can you guess what it is, well this is it. I was the first to sit in a chair which was also done by this M S, Her surname aptly summed up the ice-cold look in her eyes, S with s**** eyes. Okay, in the room were as follows – two chairs, a table, a coat or hat stand and a clock. One of these was the cause of the meeting downfall. Like a scene from a Poirot Murder Mystery, what do you think was the item in the room that upset this meeting recovery? I'll put you out of your misery, it was the clock! You see, I sat in a chair facing the only clock in the room with this lady dominatrix sitting facing me with the clock on the wall facing me but actually behind her. Then I realised during the course of the interview that she looked down several times and glanced at her wristwatch. I began to get uneasy about it as I realised that from my sitting position she could not control or time check the meeting because I controlled the clock so her only way was to look down at her watch. I soon realised that I did not matter or what I said didn't matter. Time decided both the length and the substance of my reason for being there and if time was running out, nothing I said or whatever troubled me mattered. If time was running out, I didn't matter anymore. I then quickly took control of this farce of a meeting and without any warning to her, I told her straight away that I had noticed her looking at her watch because the clock was out of view. I told her that I felt as if I was getting a watered-down, well-diluted meeting to discuss my problems. I was getting a service that was going in one ear and out the other ear. I actually felt like the lady M S did not care how the meeting went and I felt very badly let down. To me she joined my list of "fakes", but I never told her that. I did however tell her that if she had been honest with me from the beginning about everything, I would have appreciated it more. Then I stood up and told her that I was leaving as the meeting served no purpose whatsoever. This meeting and M S herself as far as I was concerned were both "fakes". It was all a fake because it was arranged as a matter of convenience. It was a procedure that had to happen for the sake of it and it made everything looked good to be part of the service. Well, it didn't work because it was timed and I had 30 minutes to get all my worries and problems off my chest, discussed and sorted. It just didn't work.

As I walked out into the waiting room, I looked at the two or three people there and I actually felt sorry for them. If they were there for the first time like me, they had no idea what was about to happen to them. I left the department and I left the building. I popped into MacDonalds for a strawberry shake and a small fries despite the metallic taste in my mouth. I spent a short time there and checked my phone for the train times to go home. After 20 minutes I made my way to London Bridge Station and got the train back to Orpington. Within an hour or so I was very quickly indoors in the warm. There truly is nothing like home. It was near 1pm and I was home in good time which for a Friday before rush hour is really, really good.

Been home now for the past hour and I suddenly feel rubbish. I am tired, weak and lost. I am alone and my God I feel alone. Loneliness is awful and to be honest is sometimes worse than the sickness. Since losing Joan, my wife and mother to Gaz, I feel empty for the first time. Then when I was told that I had cancer, my life fell apart and my life stood still. Suddenly nothing mattered but one thing I wanted to do was to get as well as possible to be able to return to my favourite place on earth which is Skiathos. I love the place and the people there. It's my little piece of paradise on this earth. I want to get better and go there again. I think and hope it will happen. It's been a long day, a day not controlled by a clock but by me taking control of the meeting by simply sitting in the wrong chair. It's time to rest and have an early night. So, before I forget it's just to let you know that disconnection of my chemo pump is due soon maybe late tomorrow or Sunday some time, I know one thing all that chemo in the balloon is now nearly all gone. All that 5FU gone into me and I got a bad feeling about next week. Things are going to get rougher now with all that chemo going in one direction into my veins and all those nooks and crannies in my body. It's Goodnight from me with more writing later or when I wake up. Cheerio all and God Bless.

——— # # # ———

GOOD MORNING, it's SATURDAY FEBRUARY 1st 2014. I was briefly sick overnight, puking up mainly water. It's now taking over me just as the chemo is taking over my body. As you know now I am taking on board very large doses of chemotherapy which is hopefully doing its work but at the same time the huge consequences are in this case resulting in me being slowly destroyed from the inside outwards. In the space of a few short weeks tom this and all because of this very cleverly created liquid chemical known as chemotherapy. My chemo is by infusion and to think that I used to be a regular blood donor with a rare blood group AB POSITIVE. (AB+). That all ended suddenly with my heart attack in 2009. Now my lovely rare blood is useless to everyone as it is contaminated by Chemotherapy. I have no idea what lies ahead, a day-to-day private battle. God it's bad now and only a few weeks in, well 4 to be exact. I have at least 14 weeks of treatment to go and I think for me the hell is only beginning. Of course I have also been told that even though the chemo infusion will end when it's meant to, the effects carry on for many, many weeks and sometimes months afterwards continuing to do those nasty horrible things to me. After all, that has to be expected as so much chemo cannot leave my system just like that. Nothing more to add today. Just to tell you that my District nurse called earlier and will be here Sunday around 7.30pm to disconnect my chemo pump which by now is a pain in the ass but hopefully doing good to me and flush my arm and PICC Line. Good night all and tomorrow is another day in this mad, mad world.

——— # # # ———

GOOD MORNING WORLD. IT'S SUNDAY FEBRUARY 2ND 2014. Today as it being Sunday means it's Mass time in St Swithun's in Fashoda Road, my usual church. My catholic faith is still strong but will be tested. I will accept this test and will not falter in any way. I will also try to go to mass as often as I can. People are praying for me but like all places there are those that remain curious and nosey and only want to see how I am reacting or suffering from the chemotherapy. Nothing pleases these clowns more than to see me having as bad a reaction as possible. As far as they are concerned, they are kept happy if they see me suffering as much as possible. Okay all, it's like this. Mass is at 10am in St Swithun's, Fashoda Road, Bromley. Mass was nice, but maybe it's because I may be getting weaker and only noticing those who mean well for me. I have to admit, I was shaken by my body behaving the way it is. I can see a big change in me now as did a lot of other people in mass today. I had a reaction from people who were visibly shaken and shocked by the change in me in these past few weeks. Just shows what chemo can do to you in such a short amount of time. Right now I can only hope that I can go to mass as often as I can, but I realise that the time will come when I will not be able to go to mass in my Church. Until then I am going to do as much as I can physically and mentally to attend mass here. I know everyone here, both genuine friends and of course my faithful fan club of fakes. I came home from mass and on the way picked up my usual paper the "Mail on Sunday", checked my lottery and did next weeks lottery. As regards the lottery, same as usual there with no wins. I then put the feet up and drifted off to sleep for the afternoon with the football on the telly in the background. I had a reasonably good day so lets not tempt fate. I took it easy. District nurse came out at 8pm, better late than never. She disconnected my chemo pump and flushed the line out, she disposed of the pump into my now clinical waste bin with my sharps bin. She done her report and left. Nothing more for me to add.

I'm feeling very sick now, more nausea than sick but hey ho! If I am being sick, I will try to write so lets see eh! I have no doubt that tonight things will change for the worse with either pain or vomiting. You know when you know your own body and all that. It is getting more difficult though this evening.

——— # # # ———

MONDAY FEBRUARY 3rd 2014 Hi all.
It is now a little after 5am and since 3.20am I have been vomiting and had diarrhoea. I have never in my life known anything like this all at the same time. It's weakening losing the liquid stomach contents from both ends of my body. Things are progressively getting worse. I know that I have to get back to bed and get some few hours sleep if I can. Goodnight...

——— # # # ———

Good morning, whatever?
Talk later or write later, I know one thing, I have to be in Guys Hospital later at 1pm, for more Chemotherapy treatment. The treatment today is not like last weeks crazy session. Today is the extra Cetuximab infusion treatment session which I hope will not be much longer than 3 or 4 hours. So not too bad I hope ... Sleep time now. ZZZZZZZZZZZZZZZZZZZZZZZZ

——— # # # ———

GOOD MORNING ALL ... It is still Monday February 3rd 2014 but at least now I got a little sleep earlier after having violent vomiting and diarrhoea. When it started, I hugged that toilet bowl and vomited into it. No sooner had I finished and gone back to bed, 5 minutes later it was all repeated again. I also notice this morning a very red inflamed rash on my neck and face. Am I worried yes I am, very, very worried. I am worried because not that it's worse than cancer but how actually bad will it become and yes, rash is on that famous list I got of the reactions that are associated with my cancer. I am aware that this has been threatening for weeks now so it's no surprise really. It's early days how bad will it get and how far will it spread throughout my entire body. I still have around 14 weeks of treatment to go and things will be bad for me for many weeks and months after that. With this happening so early it could suddenly turn me into an outcast really, really early. If not an outcast, I might find myself covering up in public places or even hiding away completely. I cannot do this.

I think I'd better contact my C N S Hannah or Claire attached to Guys and St Thomas N H S Trust. I probably know their reply but do not want to hear it. The truth can sometimes hurt. My days and nights are now gradually getting worse, a tiny bit at the time. This bloody beast of a disease is boss now and is sharing the limelight with Chemotherapy that is trying to destroy it and I'm in the middle. I don't matter any more now. One of them will win but my cancer is the aggressive type which normally is very ruthless in selecting and ultimately destroying its victims which in this case is me. Total destruction is the ultimate intention of anyone that gets in its way. I can't fight now so the chemo has to fight for me. That's it for now. Maybe tomorrow Hannah or Claire (CNS) will get back to me. Too tired now.

I just have also to let you know that I had a brief meeting with my employers in the Bus Garage this morning. It didn't last long as basically it was just a catch up and to tell them face-to-face about my cancer and my treatment. I met a lot of my work colleagues and all of them, as well as my employers representatives, were visibly shocked in how I have physically become worse since being diagnosed. It was nice however to see everyone there. The company have also agreed to carry on my sickness as long term sickness. This is what I wanted to hear from them as they have been advised officially not to "harass" any employee who is a cancer patient or even any very sick employee. I am not just a very sick employee with cancer, but an employee with a terminal illness diagnosis.

Just to explain that, after being in the Garage in New Cross, I then made my way to Guys to have my infusion of Cetuximab. It all went along as usual, and my 1pm appointment was over at 4pm and I made my way home. Another day of having a chemical pumped into me as part of the big plan. Good night all. Anyhow it cheerio from me. I will write later or tomorrow. xxx

——— # # # ———

MORNING ALL. It's Wednesday February 5th 2014 ... Yes another repeat night of vomiting, extreme tiredness and itchy red flaky skin. The skin sometimes feels like I want to scratch and scratch until it's ripped off me. This itchy flaky skin condition is new. It was red but things have progressed. Different little things now every day. There is no "bag for life", full of fun for me. God what next? It's the sickness however is the absolute worst for me now … cheerio all!

——— # # # ———

Morning all ... It is Thursday FEBRUARY 6TH 2014. How do I feel? The answer is simple. I feel very, very sick, no ending in sight. I now long for my bed every day and night. There I get some much needed rest. It shows that the chemicals are building up inside me all the time. As I looked out my bedroom window it's early morning and all the kids are on their school run. I look out at them and think of them and their future. I have lived on this road since 2004 and I know a lot of these kids and their parents. It saddens me that with my diagnosis, I may not be alive to see these kids grow up and complete their education in our local school. Then I think when I was a child back in Ireland and it really does not matter what country you are from when you are a child, cancer does not bother you normally and then without any warning you are struck down with it. As a child or a young adult, you may not even notice cancer in your life but as I look at these young school kids, I think that one day there is a high possibility that at least one or two of them will be struck down with cancer and some of the others may be considering further education in Oncology, Consultants, GPs and nurses. Then there are the tiny minority of those who even when they are adults have no idea or opinion on cancer. This is of course based on cancer nowadays however in years to come that may not be the case as it is predicted that cancer will be hitting or affect in one way or another every single person on this earth. Absolutely nobody on earth will escape the clutches of cancer. It is a very sad fact that this will happen despite all the damn money being pumped into cures for cancer. As I look out the same window these kids are full of life not a care in the world, nothing bothering them. God it would be so nice if this did not change. As I still look out the same bedroom window, I feel the radiator in the room up full and lately I'm needing all the heat in the world. My body is having it's condition deteriorating so quickly now that my heating is on both night and day. My body is shaking, shivering with the cold and it's cold because the chemotherapy chemicals are killing the cells in my body every minute of every day now. I have so many weeks to go yet and I really cannot see me doing this. It is terrible, absolutely awful and I am totally unprepared for this. All the leaflets and the consultants advice in the beginning is nothing compared to the real thing. Please do not Google or You Tube your cancer or your treatment as it is nothing like it. It also makes it worse. What happens when you get to see or hear what it says on those websites can be totally wrong. Don't get me wrong, some are correct and some are not but it's the wrong info ones that mess you up. The best thing is to get actual proper physical advice from your consultant or your CNS, absolutely nobody else. That's it today. Tomorrow is another day. Please God I will wake up after my sleep and get through another day. Good night all. ZZZZZZZZZZZZ.

——— # # # ———

Morning all. It's Friday February 7th 2014 and now things are playing games with me and my head. The rash that was annoying me is now easing a little and I think it's because I havent had the 3 chemo drugs in a while. Last week I just had the one Cetuximab so maybe at this stage the build up of drugs is not enough to cause any extra symptoms of rash. I have no doubt that in the coming weeks things will result in some form of inflammation or rash. To think overall today, eased rash and feeling relatively good, it might be a good weekend after all. Just had a lovely chat with Gaz, now there is one hell of a strong person. I take all my strength from him. I will do all in my power to stay around for Gaz for a long, long time. If I have to say this every day I will, but I love this boy of mine so much. I will close while I am good, bring on the weekend all of it. Time to rest this body now and go back to bed. Good day to all of you. Tomorrow is Saturday February 8th. 2014

——— # # # ———

GOOD MORNING ALL. SATURDAY FEBRUARY 8th 2014. Yeah, too good to be true. Woke up with a face full of terrible rash. Beats me why it returned, but it has really ruined my weekend good and proper. Sorry am going back to bed after taking on some fluids. No mood to eat now. Also no vomiting today, then again nothing eaten so nothing to come up and the anti-sickness is doing its work. I have decided to go back to bed and cancel the rest of today. Tomorrow is Saturday 8th.

——— # # # ———

GOOD MORNING ALL. It is Sunday February 9th 2014. Was very sick overnight. Didnt expect that at all as I was prepared for a quiet one. Regret to say that I cannot do mass today so staying in bed for most of today. Therefore I am staying upstairs. Maybe I will just lay on the bed, go through my phone again and again. I don't know how many times I have noticed this but if I put my phone down and pick it up within a minute and open up my Facebook, there is always something new on it. Right now I spend my life on Facebook. Right back to earth and back to bed. I have a funny feeling that I am going to see an awful lot of this bed of mine. It's a fall back but it's a damn good one. If I could move my entire life and all the important things in life to have beside me then I would have them beside my bed. Already so many people have told me that as the treatment progresses, my bed will become the focal point of my cancer, it's treatment, recovery and final getting back to some form of being normal. My consultant Theresa has told me that my cancer is aggressive, sneaky and controlling. She told me it will be possible to notice that it will change places, hide and disappear in one place and in a scan will pop up elsewhere. So right now let me take this in hand and let the rest of today go by. I am going to my bed and get up hopefully not overnight vomiting but in the morning, like a normal, sick, morning vomiting person, if there is such a thing as normal vomiting. Tomorrow I am back in Guys Hospital for another dose of that drug CETUXIMAB. I am getting to like Cetuximab or maybe getting used to it should be the correct way of saying it. I suppose it's a way of my mind saying that I am getting accustomed to it. Theresa calls it the "extra help drug" and she has a lot of faith in this drug, so bring on the Cetuximab and if it helps. My God, I am going to be so, so happy if it works and get me my extension to life. So Goodnight. I said this ages ago and am saying it again tonight last time. Goodnight and God Bless xx

——— # # # ———

MORNING ALL, it is Monday February 10th 2014. No vomiting last night or this morning. It cannot last, I know it won't. Time for a shower and a nice shave. My appointment today on the 10th floor Cancer Day Unit is at 3pm. I feel a bit rough but nothing that a spoonful of anti-sickness medicine can't cure. Just had a spoonful and it's horrible, bloody horrible clear liquid. All bloody weird with my metallic taste and the anti-sickness tastes horrible like it should do. Just when I wanted something tasting metallic it bloody lets me down and tastes rubbish ... can't win can I. Still feel okay and it's near 1.30pm and time to do that trek up to Guys. Cab is due any minute. Had a good chat with the cab driver from Cannon Cars and as I already knew, cancer is now everywhere. He told me his family are plagued with cancer incidents. I don't know if he said it to feel sorry for me or not but who knows. But it is true that more and more people are getting cancer nowadays. Met Peter who I know in Orpington Station and got the train to Guys. Arrived in Guys with plenty of time to spare. On the way got my large fries and strawberry shake but it tasted disgustingly metallic. I ate it as it was all I would or could eat today. My taste buds are getting gradually worse and disappearing. I didn't finish the fries and shake. I went into Guys and took a seat in the lobby after getting a rip off cup of tea. It was about 2.40pm so to allow at least 5 minutes or so to get to the 10th floor, I had 15 minutes here to watch the world go by. In here is a different world going by. The main entrance has 2 revolving doors. Just outside these doors is a normal world. I say normal but normal life goes on but the world goes by.

On the road outside Guys, people walk or run past, but there is a divide. Picture the scene, people meandering along, going about their business, then at times you suddenly see groups of people or individuals drift away from their line of walking and turn in towards the hospital. This is the great divide, but there is still a mix of sick and healthy. Through those doors into the foyer of the hospital, on one side to the right is the information desk and on the other side is the cafe and snacks where you literally take out the equivalent of a small mortgage for a coffee and a cupcake. Ask for a toasted sandwich is good but to pay for it and it's enough to trigger a mild heart attack. At the information desk, the direction info leaflets are stacked up. Also here is a human being that will tell you on request where the various departments are, but still it is human nature to actually pick up a leaflet or a hospital info map. Is it any wonder how hundreds of leaflets disappear on a daily basis. I sat and watched the world go by and then, in the space of only 15 minutes that I was there, I began to recognise faces. That is when you know that the hospital and its people are now a part of your life and in some cases peoples final months of life. I thought to myself, how many people are here today to get a prognosis on their scans etc? Then I thought of all the people who came through those revolving doors today in a neutral state of mind. How many would leave through these same doors with a sentence of death hanging over them? I watched that door transfixed of all the people going in and out. Eventually my time was up and then I realised that so many of these people are doctors and nurses going in and out and the same "laws of health" also applies to them. Yes, the "laws of health" applies to everyone. We are all in the same boat and some of these boats will sink and some will float. Anyhow, I took the lift to the 10th floor and went into the Cancer Day Unit. After a few minutes in the queue to check in, I gave my details and my appointment card was taken and exchanged for a wristband like as I said before all inclusive chemotherapy but today is one drug infusion of

Cetuximab so I don't get my moneys worth of chemicals. Theresa believes in this Cetuximab so I will take this one drug anytime but as things are going at the moment, I am actually getting Cetuximab every week now. Week 1 with two other drugs and then as well on week 2 and week 3. After a blood test I had to wait an hour and was then called in. I was seen at 4.20pm in Cubicle B, right in the corner. I made myself comfortable and awaited my needles etc. All were connected in a few minutes and opposite me today was a lady resembling a jockey. Like I said before, these are patients wearing helmets with flowing cold water to prevent the hair loss during chemotherapy treatment. It however is not for me. I fell asleep feet up which was so relaxing. At a little after 6.30pm, one of the nurses woke me up. She disconnected my Cetuximab and gave me time to recover before getting my appointment card for the next appointment. I stood up and felt dizzy. I was then aware that I had not taken any water while I was there for the 3 hours or so. I was never one to take on loads of water and today was no exception. I went to the loo and sure enough my urine was very bright yellow nearly orange, a sure sign of no water in my system. I drank quite a lot of water and then left to go to the lift which eventually led to the ground floor and out the main entrance of Guys and then onto London Bridge Station. It was around 7.15pm and the mad rush was over but I was glad to get home and indoors into the warmth and comfort of my home. It was late but I had a bowl of soup that tasted horrible like metal. Yes I had that metallic taste in my mouth. Earlier this morning it was a bland taste of paper. Now it was full blown metallic taste. I was told in the beginning it was on the list of reactions to my chemo treatment. However it is only 39 days since I started chemo and now this is happening more and more. I still have at least 14 or 15 weeks to go and the worst is yet to come. Hair loss has still not happened, if it will happen. I havent got a lot of it anyway but will I have any less, I still don't know. That's it for today, TV time and bed. No idea about later but as the chemo builds up, vomiting later is a huge possibility… Lets see eh! Goodnight all...

——— # # # ———

Good Morning all … it's Tuesday February 11th 2014 and it is just after 7am. Yes, I have also just puked my guts up. It was nothing like normal vomiting but was more like pure angry, stomach wrenching, painful violent puking, the kind that made me sweat and left me sitting on the toilet floor breathless. Never had anything like it so things are really happening now. Okay. it's 9.20am and just been puking up again only water as there is nothing else in there. I havent got the energy to shave today but I ask myself, who the hell is going to see me. I certainly am not going out anywhere as I expect a day hugging the toilet bowl on and off. Anyhow some Domperidone anti-sickness might help. Bloody hell, what a day and been getting sick yet again on and off despite the anti-sickness medicine. Now I am sick to high hell of the anti-sickness. That's it Goodnight all, been a terrible day and need to rest now and an early night again.

——— # # # ———

Hi all. WEDNESDAY FEBRUARY 12th 2014. Quiet night, no sick yet but I have noticed a slight weight loss. It has to be expected as I have not eaten much recently because of this metallic taste in my mouth. I need to increase my water drinking though. Like a lot of people, I do not take in a lot of water or should I say enough water. It is bad for me tiredness and headaches. It's afternoon now and just been lying on the bed so going to take an easy evening now and just do a little reading. Next Monday is the triple Chemotherapy hit. Goodnight all.

——— # # # ———

THURSDAY FEBRUARY 13TH 2014 ... Hi all, it is one hell of a crap day already. I can't take much more of it. I am tired, no energy, sick, headaches and that slight rash of recent times is back this morning. No doubt now, no doubt whatsoever about it now, the chemotherapy is building up in my body and it is hurting a lot. Sorry, I need to go, this is too much. Sick of it all ...FRIDAY, FEBRUARY 14TH 2014 ... SATURDAY FEBRUARY 15TH 2014... SUNDAY FEBRUARY 16TH 2014...

——— # # # ———

MONDAY FEBRUARY 17TH 2014 Morning all.
Sorry. I am so, so sorry but it has been pure uncensored almighty hell. I realise that I have been quite for a few days, sorry more than that. Bloody hell, last Thursday was when I wrote last and today is Monday. Well here goes. All I did on Friday, Saturday and Sunday was vomit, vomit, vomit, sweat, cry, sweat, scream to myself more vomit, scream and think. Thinking is dangerous on your own. I was thinking on my own and I came up with ideas, questions and solutions but the conclusion was the same. I have bloody cancer and I am sick and there is every possibility that I may die sometime in the next 16 months. Like I said, thinking is dangerous so it's best never to be alone when this shit is going on. I have Garreth (Gaz), family, good friends and neighbours so please, please do not ever be alone if you are going through a similar situation. I cannot stress this point enough. It's bad, its awful for me or anybody to be struck down with cancer. Treatment and recovery is hell, but if the treatment does not work, it is the worst place in the world for anybody dealing with it both patient and anybody caring for the patient. In my case its only a matter of weeks into my journey. Who knows where the journey will go from here, but here I go. Right

then, today is 3 Chemotherapy drugs time again. Yes the All Inclusive version, wrist bands and all that. It all happens for me in Guys later at 10.30 this morning. Early treatment usually means there for the next 6 to maybe 7 hours treatment for a 3 drug infusion session of Cisplatin, 5FU and Cetuximab with in between infusion of various fluids including Piriton which makes me sleepy and relaxed for the whole thing to happen. Then I will have a pump then connected to me 24/4. I may have said in the past about this as going into me 24/7, of course I meant 24/4 as it is going into me over a period of 4 days and not 7 therefore 24/4. The usual thing happened. I got the train from Orpington to London Bridge, walked down the usual slope from the platform into the station. I walked past the beggars and the preachers and leaflet distributors, past MacDonalds and left into the hospital through the revolving doors, past the coffee and snacks into the lift to the 10th floor and the Cancer Day Unit. There, at the desk, I exchanged my appointment card for the all inclusive wristband. No waiting around today. No blood test as I was taken straight to my cubicle in a zone. It was all happening quickly today which is what I needed today. Gaz came down around 2pm. I love that boy so much with what he is going through right now with me. After Gaz had gone back to work, I started drifting off to sleep again. All the treatments went ahead as usual. I did manage to get my pump attached and after collecting my appointment card for next week, I left the usual way via lift and foyer to the Station. I needed to get out of here reasonably early as it will be an early night etc. I was pleased that it did all go well and my pump was connected and I have an early start as I need to be in Luton Airport for a flight to Varna in Bulgaria and then a long drive to Razgrad as that is where Milena is living. I realise that as my treatment progresses, I may get too sick an all that to keep up the travelling to Bulgaria. With the situation today, I have to be back here on Friday as my district nurse is disconnecting on Saturday this time. Okay all, after getting home its time for that reasonably early bedtime and that early morning trip to Luton and then to Varna, if possible. Again, also in the back of my mind is that ultimately with my chemo building up and therefore maybe unable to travel to Milena in Bulgaria, our relationship may suffer badly. Anyhow moving on. Goodnight all and I will write tomorrow even though I have a lot going on right now.

——— # # # ———

Good Morning all, I have to get straight to the point. It's Tuesday February 18th 2014, it's early morning and I feel like shit... I gotta take it easy as I need to get to Luton Airport, fly to Varna and meet Milena after a drive to Razgrad. I took the whole thing in my stride, all easy going. Deep down I think it's a futile attempt to avoid being alone in life. I met Milena last Summer in Skiathos in Greece. I have been going there on holiday since the 1980s. I met Milena there as she goes there to work and she worked in my apartments cleaning etc. I was alone and we met or as I now believe, we didn't meet, more like I was selected? Whatever happens, I will not leave home to live in Bulgaria, never. My son Garreth is here and I promise him now I will never leave his side to live in any other country. I promise that to Gaz now and even though it all seems exciting and gives me a purpose to carry on and get better, but I know that also I may get too sick to continue these trips to see Milena out in Bulgaria. Everything in Bulgaria is so far behind what we have in England. My God, what will I do if that sickness comes sooner rather than later. Anyhow right now I'm in Razgrad but back home again in a couple of days. This evening I am in Razgrad in a Pizza Restaurant called The Crazy Forest and then it dawned on me that I don't know Bulgarian and Milena doesn't know any English. I had my google translator and it is slow and I knew then that this was not going to work out for the better. I had a long road ahead of me at home and was determined to make the most of this different but possibly temporary relationship with Milena. Just like my whole life, I looked around me and I was a complete stranger here. My life in fact was just like what it is around me right now this evening. It is late in the evening and look what happens in the evening where the setting sun casts shadows as it sets, is possibly where my life is going right now. Like my life and the setting sun all makes. As I look at all my pain and torment physically and mentally compared to actually having cancer, at the moment the treatment is worse than the cancer diagnosis, so bad in fact that dying is in fact the easy bit! ... My day and for all I know my life is drawing to a close. Yes I have a chemotherapy pump so flying here actually had my chemo going into me at over 400mph, yes speedy chemo. Okay all, I bid you goodnight. GOODNIGHT xx

——— # # # ———

GOOD MORNING EVERYONE, and it's Wednesday February 19th 2014. Yes, it's good morning from Razgrad in Bulgaria. If this was The Eurovision Song Contest my next line would be "and here are the votes from the Bulgarian jury", but it's not. It is morning and it is cold here and my health is awful this morning. I have been getting sick and I feel tired and to be honest I will not be doing this on a regular basis like this. Also I feel more comfortable back in the UK where the health system is no comparison. Bulgaria is too basic for my disease, so Friday home will in fact be a blessing when it comes. In the meantime this trip is a relaxing one or at least it's meant to be. I fly to Varna from Luton Airport. In Varna I hire a car and then drive for one and a half hours to Razgrad. Varna is a really beautiful airport but the road to Razgrad is shall we say, interesting! This road is also the main road to Ruse via Schumen. Most of it is two or three lanes wide in each direction and is of good quality. However, there is no street lighting on 80% of the road. The worst part is the part from Varna Airport to the turn off for Schumen. On the way to Razgrad I drive through sleepy little villages whose names I cannot pronounce but it is clearly obvious that I am in Eastern Europe and it is so blatantly obvious that the people are very, very poor. One thing I must say is that I thoroughly enjoy driving on this road from Varna Airport to Razgrad. Because of my flight times, my journey on this road is nearly always in the dark. The return however is nearly always in daylight. Let me tell you now that, from what I have seen, a combination of poor road lighting, poor driver abilities, excessive speed and reckless driving leads to a lethal mix with terrible consequences. I have not been driving on this road for long but already I have seen the aftermath of some awful accidents involving a lot of vehicles. On Tuesday night on the way here I came across 3 such accidents on the way to Razgrad. Yes, I had a near miss on a part that was a dark, 2 lane motorway near Beli Lom Lake. I was doing 70kph in the dark when out of nowhere appeared a herd of 10 to 12 cattle and 2 dogs, no humans with them so I assume they escaped from a nearby farm or field. I only saw them at the last minute and it scared the hell out of me. Lucky I was careful on a new strange road. Bulgaria is different and nice but as I already said, I know that I cannot live here. For the benefit of you knowing about my health here, I took it easy and it will end on Friday and I can return home. Anyhow on Saturday I am expecting a district nurse to disconnect my chemo pump and flush the PICC Line out properly. Here in Razgrad that pump has been awkward and I have been sick but for some reason even though I feel bad sometimes, it's been mild so far. I now hope that nothing bad happens to my condition while I am here in Bulgaria. By now it is obvious that the chemo is building up in my body and drastic changes to my body, both inside and outside are happening. Anyhow it's the end of another day here in Razgrad. I am spending the next few hours here with Milena, her son Denis, her friend Galya. Also here is her daughter Gergana (Geri), and her son Teddy and partner Pavlin. Lovely family who really are over the top with family love and so much hospitality. It is late in the day and the evening shadows lengthen let me say Goodnight to you all. GOODNIGHT XX

——— # # # ———

Morning to you all. It is THURSDAY FEBRUARY 20TH 2014. Another day in Razgrad and it's home time tomorrow. Finally I do feel rough today and to be honest, I was wondering if I was actually going to get sick or not any more than normal. Well I got my answer. Yes I do have all my medication here with me and I am using them. I am staying here in the Hotel Central and today is my last full day and Milena, Denis her son and I are off to the Ludogorets Football Club and training ground. Later we are going to their actual stadium.

Getting very tired already this morning so I will close. You don't really want to know the grotty details what I get up to. I will write tomorrow before I leave Razgrad and Milena. The problem is that every time here now could also be my last. My condition changes every hour and day now so who knows if or when I will be here again. Goodnight all xx

——— # # # ———

Good Morning all, it is FRIDAY FEBRUARY 21ST 2014. I left Milena's family very late last night. Her family did lay out a lot of food and drink but I could not take a chance especially on my last day here, so I did hold back on the booze especially. Also, I have a gastric band with medium restriction so that actually helped me to hold back. I used to be over 24 stone until a heart attack in 2007 changed my life. I also smoked and therefore probably the reason why I have this bloody cancer now. Anyhow after a 2 year waiting, I had my gastric band in may 2009 and am now just over 12 stone in weight. Okay back to Razgrad etc, last night for the first time ever I ate horse meat. It tasted okay but I will not be repeating the experience, ever again. I am in enough trouble with cancer so am not in a mood to be ending up having any horse meat reactions like jumping fences, eating hay or even doing a poo while I walk. After taking Milena home, I got back to the hotel late. She is at work this morning and when she finishes at lunchtime, we have a few hours together before I leave to drive to Varna airport. I will write again at the airport...

Okay all, here I am in Varna Airport. It did hurt me to leave Milena but I have my treatment to get through and what goes with it. Yes, I cried leaving Razgrad and did so for the next 30 to 40 minutes on that road to Varna Airport. My flight is in 1 hour and 10 minutes time. I am through security waiting for that flight after 7pm. I miss Milena a lot. I also feel very tired and now have a new thing, I have leg cramps from that drive from Razgrad to the Airport at least I can rest on the flight which is around 2 hours and 50 minutes I think. No more writing today now while I take it easy and get home I will write sometime tomorrow again...

——— # # # ———

GOOD MORNING ALL, It is SATURDAY FEBRUARY 22ND 2014 and it's a new day for me. Back home and yes of course missing Milena terribly. Overnight with all the upset of getting back and things going through my mind, I felt sick. The anti-sickness did work for a while but from 2am onwards I was very, very sick for an hour and a half hanging over the toilet bowl. Not sick in Razgrad, I get home and get sick. Well, whats done is done. Tonight the pump is being disconnected so it's obvious that the chemicals are building up in my body and I am half expecting all hell to break lose very, very soon inside and outside my body. It has been too quiet for too long now so it is well overdue. The district nurse arrived just after 8pm. She noted in her report all that she done. In her report it looked like she was here for hours, shall we say creating work that was not needed nor was it done. Fiction work! She disconnected that hideous grey package of a pump with its clear liquid chemo inside a balloon which was hanging over my shoulder sideways. It does as you know by now resemble a slowly deflating balloon as the 4 days or so goes by. It was fitted late on Monday night and I wore it on Tuesday, Wednesday, Thursday and Friday. The balloon was actually empty this morning so it was okay to have it removed tonight. I am now free of it until a repeat in three weeks time. It was flushed out tonight with saline and cleaned and dressed the area where the connection to the blood supply is in my upper left arm. It is then tucked away neatly, dressed, protected and securely covered with an elasticated dressing patch. I have a couple of these elasticated bandages as I have to sometimes now wash and dry my own from time to time. The nurse did eventually leave, she really couldn't get out quick enough. No time to spare is what she said, too many other visits, no time to chat at all. I then simply watched TV and had an early night. Just before bedtime I did notice redness in face and neck. I intend to take a closer look in the morning. I hope to have a reasonably quiet night. I am going to take some anti-sickness now just as a precaution rather than anything else, Good night all. God willing, I will be here in the morning. I did say that things will go downhill sooner rather than later. Good night all and will write in the morning if I can.

——— # # # ———

GOOD MORNING ALL, it's SUNDAY FEBRUARY 23RD 2014 and maybe it is not for discussion but I just had a vomiting session. Things have progressed, the rash is now a bright redness all over my neck and face. I feel like crap, I am tired and very weak. This is gradually going to get worse now. Back to bed now and get some rest. It is now 8.20am and I have just been violently vomiting again. It didn't last long at all but all the time in Bulgaria was very little and now, well it's all the time. I wish now that Milena and her family had seen me at my worst. Just to see the effort that I am putting in to keep in contact with Milena while sick and I still travelled. Then I thought, I need the break away to escape the hell with this cancer and the surroundings of cancer. I sometimes wonder if it was it good to meet Milena or not, but I did meet her and for what it's worth, it's good. One thing that does bother me however is that I do have annoying moments when I sit in restaurants and bars in silence because of the language barrier. I say now that surely it will not last a year for Milena and I. For now I am back home and back to reality, I am sick and have no immediate plans to go back to Razgrad. My treatment plans and reactions will decide this. I am not going back to bed again today but maybe lie downstairs on the couch or armchair. While up I have to make the most of today. I cannot go to mass today for the simple reason that, as of now, this very moment, I feel awful, tired and this large area of redness on my face and neck is embarrassing and making me feel annoyed and upset by my appearance in a public place like at church, and more so as I know most of these people who have not seen me as bad as this ever before.

It is forcing me to stay out of the public view, well for today at least. I dare say that things may get bad enough now for me that I may not see my church for a long time now. Tomorrow is back to Guys for an infusion of one drug CETUXIMAB at 11am ... Change of plan, I have just decided to take my anti-sickness and brave it out and go to Mass at 10am. I will be shut away for long enough, avoiding people long enough, time to face the music, or the hymns! I need to maintain my religion which is important to me. When I think about it, I only maintain my religion and the people nearest and dearest to me.

I am now out of mass. I got there early. My usual friends are here, John and Jackie, my elderly but lovely friend Anne. John and Jackie love their holidays and especially their cruises. I have an ongoing joke with John that I already shared with you that as he sits on the seat edge and ever since I saw him get splashed one day with holy water, I told him in future bring an umbrella to church and it reminds him of being splashed by a wave on his cruise. When the priest does the blessing of the churchgoers with the holy water, John always gets splashed and always has the water marks on his glasses to prove it. Anne lost her husband a few years ago, an Italian man he was and she is so quiet and leads a simple life. We will be friends for life. Then there is Sandra and Mark, Mary S and her son, John and Betty D, Rosemary and David who live for part of the year on the other side of the world. Ada is here with her two young kids, she lost her husband last year. Another friend of mine is Pearl C, very old and very, very frail but still gets out as much as she can. Because Pearl sits on the top of the church seats, when I go up to receive holy communion, I touch Pearls shoulder and she reaches out to grab my hand. She was devastated when she heard first that I had cancer. There are so many people in this church that I know, like my other family. During the mass service I look up to the top of the church and I realise that it is here that my coffin will be on supports when I die from this cancer or something else. It was here that I had the funeral for my wife Joan in 2008. If the cancer has its way, I will be here in 18 months or so from now if the cancer wins, however, the idea is that it will not win. I have to delay it for as long as possible. After mass, it's home time and feet up for the rest of the day. I get home, had a mug of tea and 5 minutes later I took my medication. It's now a little after 12 noon and I feel a little sick. Ten to fifteen minutes later and I was hugging the toilet bowl upstairs and started vomiting violently. It was then that I noticed a strange smell but cannot tell what it is. Maybe it is something new that will show its face later on if not sooner but I can't help notice that I have smelled it before. It's in the toilet but there's something else that is not quite yet showing its face to me. More surprises I'm sure in store for me....

Well, I survived the day, still feel wretched from the earlier vomiting. I really do feel tired and that bright red rash on my face and neck has now extended down to my chest area. I am now taking Doxycycline capsules for it. I was given these a few weeks ago in preparation for when I get this rash. Now that the rash is here and establishing itself I am taking this medication. I fear however that it is not going to be enough as my 3 chemo drugs are in all very high doses and then the pump attached 24/4 may altogether be too much for the DOXYCYCLINE to cope and keep it controlled. I need to see my GP again soon for something stronger to control it. Okay all you lovely people out there, I am taking the rest of the day to relax. I will write tomorrow morning if I can when I wake up. I have an early start tomorrow as even though it is up to Guys for 11am chemo appointment and an early start usually means there all day. Tomorrow is different in that it is only one chemotherapy drug infusion. Good night all.

——— # # # ———

GOOD MORNING ALL ...
It is MONDAY February 24th 2014, I got up twice during the night and had the two vomiting sessions. No sign of any improvement in the rash but maybe it's early days and for all I know nothing will happen until all my treatment is over. I am now also using Double base Gel as of this morning for moisturising. I have also just taken a load of Domperidone anti-sickness liquid. That and most other things are now all tasting more metallic but can you believe it, the anti-sickness tastes exactly as it is and not metallic or like paper. It tastes disgusting as it is. Right, I gotta get my ass in gear and get ready, my chemo appointment for infusion is in its usual place in Guys at 11am. I have to get to Orpington Station and my usual train to London Bridge Station. The Monday routine is the same now as before. Cab for 9.45am, then a train after 10am. One thing I have noticed this morning is a slight touch of fatigue creeping in now. It's barely noticeable, but to me when it's new it's different and now I'm always on the lookout for different changes to me and my body. It is the same for everyone, you always know your own body and any of its changes no matter how small or big they are. I don't know if I explained this or not but let me again explain how I am doing this book. For many years now going back a long time, I updated a diary every day for work. Being a bus driver and all that it entailed/needed me to record in writing the day in a diary. Of course, when I

was diagnosed it was so obvious to write even more and in more detail. Now here I am converting it to the form of a book and in the shape of a daily blog. My style of writing technique is as plain and simple as possible so most people can read it, understand it and take it in. I apologise also for the way my language and ways of getting a message across to you is or appears poor or different. I write about something as I say it or as I see it and describe it. I have no idea how many books are on the market about dealing with cancer, but this is my one and it's about my journey. I only want good to come out of it. I also realise that some days may appear dramatic and some days nothing at all is written. If I write nothing it only means that nothing actually happened or I may be too sick to write. It is what it is and there you go, I did it again, I diverted away from the matter on hand, nobodys fault, just mine. I am tired more than ever today and that smell I am noticing again in the toilet, I noticed it again this morning. I still can't put my finger on it, but the cause of it will come to me. It has to be new as it is only since my illness began. It's annoying me now and I will find the cause very soon. Anyhow, a train trip up here and down the ramp at London Bridge. Then, it's along the area under the train track and out near the street that leads to the entrance to the Hospital. It's 10.45am and soon I am on the 10th floor and in The Cancer Day Unit.

The way down here involved the usual Monday treatment of the public rushing about and knocking against each other. This is my usual routine straight from London Bridge Station and no stopping until I get to those revolving doors at the entrance to Guys' Hospital. No stopping today for the large fries and vanilla shake because now it all taste disgusting and metallic. Inside the hospital revolving doors at the entrance, there are the usual queues for coffee, teas and snacks, even fruit. Other people just sitting there and watching the world go by and probably people watching other people and in their own minds making up their own series of diagnosis of complete strangers just by looking at them. It is all pure innocent fun and passes the time with fun. Of course I do the same but at a distance like before I pick out the male doctors etc, just by what they wear. If a bloke has a light coloured shirt, light or chords trousers and a pair of brown or hush puppies type shoes then he is a doctor or consultant. However the Stethoscope around the neck or hanging out the pocket is a dead giveaway. Up here in the Cancer Day Unit today, Richard and Evelyn are on the front desk with Heena again in the office. The door to Heena's office is shut, that means stay away she is too busy to chat. I hand over my appointment card and in return I get my All Inclusive chemotherapy wrist band, then I sit and wait. I smile politely at the other people in the waiting room and slowly I can now tell, yes even this early in my treatment, the difference between those cursed by this disease and those who are involved in the care of the patients. Cancer patients are cursed, cursed by fate but still lucky to have the lifeline of treatment in a place like this. Every day I think to myself. People born 50 years from now will probably find that cancer will be almost non existant. Which one would I prefer? I still don't know the answer to that one.... Suddenly I was called for a blood test. I already know that it will take an hour to get results back from the lab, that means a delay in treatment as nothing ever goes ahead until results are back. It is now 11.07am so no treatment at least until after 12 noon to 12.15pm. After the blood test I returned to the waiting area but soon realised that I had lost my seat. Many of those seated were looking very healthy and were there to look after cancer patients but still none of them offered me a seat. I suppose that I wasn't looking sick enough to be offered a seat. Maybe that's good and if it is the case then in a matter of weeks I will be looking sick and tired etc then I will have no trouble in getting offered a seat. If that's the case, then I can wait. At 12.25pm without anybody offering me a seat, I was called into Cubicle 8 in Zone C.... One day Cetuximab treatment today and I should be finished in about 3 hours or so from now. That gets me out of here between 3.30 and 4.00pm and still getting a train before rush hour kicks in. I dread rush hour. Not many people like rush hour anyway. Gaz came down to be with me for an hour or so during his lunch break as he always does. He has a lot on his plate with work etc but he still pops down to visit me while I'm all connected up via my PICC line. As usual during the treatment, they gave me Piriton which makes me sleepy always. I soon obliged the instructions and fell asleep to dream. Obviously my blood levels were good and my full treatment went ahead after my wristband details were checked and all until the last bag of Cetuximab was going up. I woke up around 3pm and the bag of Cetuximab was nearly empty. Once it was empty, one of the nurses flushed the line out with saline when all was disconnected. I said my goodbyes, got my appointment card and left.

I went straight downstairs and out of the hospital and headed straight for London Bridge Station. My journey from the hospital lift took me past all those in the foyer people watching and like me diagnosing peoples diseases just by observations from a distance, past all the doctors and nurses in the coffee queue. I again thought to myself that there's nobody on the wards as theyre all down here with lighted cigarettes in one hand and pushing connected up packs of fluid on drip trolleys in the other hand. I then brushed past the beggars and the Jehovah Witnesses with their have a lovely day messages near MacDonalds. I went up the escalator past the guys in Black Overcoats as Shard security and past that open air freezing part of the London Bridge area. Platform 1 has a train in 7 minutes I think, even though I am tired, I should make it. By the time I got to Platform 1, I was wiped out totally and absolutely exhausted now. Look how quick this fatigue came over me. The train was quiet and from the station I took a taxi home. At home I secured the house, took some fluids on board and went to bed. I awaited an anxious night of nausea and probably vomiting was almost guaranteed to be ahead of me. It was only 5.20pm but after going to the loo, it had to be bed. GOOD NIGHT all and I will try to write again later or tomorrow...

——— # # # ———

GOOD MORNING EVERYONE. It is TUESDAY FEBRUARY 25th 2014. Before I went to bed last night I tried to explain that I was very tired but having problems passing urine. I will explain now here but first let me tell you that even though I was vomiting slightly but not on a huge scale, I will now try to explain that now even passing urine is just starting to be a little different when I say different, I mean different. It's beginning to concern me slightly that lately it is taking me longer to now pass urine. Without too much detail, I just stand there and it takes a lot of time to now pass urine. Yes, it is on the list of symptoms, but I never expected it to take effect so soon into my treatment. My team in Guys gave me a list of treatment symptoms like a family tree. So many things will happen, so many symptoms, but as the list goes on, the list actually branches off as the symptoms show themselves and then you find yourself with another list branching off. Let me explain something, so far things have happened and as my cancer is Head and Neck Cancer, that is the location of the primary source near my throat at base of my tongue and near a tonsil, and that they tell me has grown back. In that spot created a cancerous tumour. The chemotherapy created further reactions and symptoms that can go in any direction. On the list is a reaction concerning hearing. If I have hearing problems, then we go on further down the list. If not, then we divert away on a totally different route. In my case my hearing was not affected so we avoided going in that direction and concentrated on going the other way. So now as we are on that other direction, we will be looking for symptoms on that direction and so on and so forth. As the treatment progresses, I found out it diverts again two ways, hair loss and no hair loss. Mine is no hair loss so that will be my symptom list direction and as it continues it will again be divided and sub divided and sub divided again. Each cancer is different as is each type of treatment and reaction to treatment. Chemotherapy is truly absolutely awful and as my treatment progresses, it will take its toll on me and destroy my mind and body. It will destroy me as a person. It is destroying me now and will continue to destroy me until there will be nothing left of me to resemble a human being. I do not know the outcome if I survive or not. It is 8pm only but I have to stop here as I have to do some other work quickly. I have to complete my Personal Independence Payment application. I will post it tomorrow. I must also apply for my Employment Support Allowance and post that tomorrow. If all is successful then I will have a Blue Badge, as one comes with the other. Sorry, I must stop and close for now. I will try to write later and explain but It may be tomorrow as I suddenly feel very low and lonely and sad on the inside. GOODNIGHT ALL.

——— # # # ———

GOOD MORNING TO YOU ALL. It is Wednesday February 26th 2014. When I stopped writing last night about 8pm or so and I had intended to come back to write but I couldn't. I tried but let me tell you that for the first time ever I cried and cried out loud. Sometimes I screamed and wanted to die there and then. I hated everyone healthy out there, yes everyone. I hated the doctors and nurses treating me yet if they were sick, who would help me. The answer is simple, no one. There would be no one to help me. I am sorry for hating the doctors and nurses, it's how my mind is reacting. In actual fact, I love the doctors and nurses. I think this is the first time that things have got to me like this and now I hate myself even more for thinking like this. Also, for the first time I nearly stopped feeling positive and for a few seconds maybe I got that scary feeling in that I would be better off if I died now. Yes, it's a horrible thought but there you go, I'm holding nothing back here. If it's on my mind then I'm going to put it on paper and it's guaranteed that if you are reading this and considered all that I have said then there is always the possibility of maybe you contemplating suicide. Nobody wants to admit it but the probability is there then. It will be in your mind, as it's in mine and it is nothing to be ashamed of. Never ever bloody forget one thing, it is normal to feel this way and do not let anyone try to change your mind. Do not let people control how you feel, they have absolutely no idea how you feel or what youre going through. People may step back and act strange by how you feel and may appear shocked or upset, then f*** them, they are not true friends. True friends will accept without question all you say and do. You're the one with the cancer and if it puts them out, so be it. I know now and anyone reading this knows that as soon as you get cancer, you are no longer in charge. Cancer is boss now. The Cancer has selected you like an Alien. You are the host and it is now in charge of you. Take my case for example, Cancer has selected me to be a host. Being a host is, in this case, a shit job but it's life. As a host, I am at its mercy. The Cancer will do all it can to stay with me. It likes its new home inside me and if at all possible it will pay visits to other parts of my body to view my other internal organs as a second or third or even more of a home. How? Well, like me in the Cancer Day Centre all inclusive. Cancer too has an imaginary wrist band and it hitches a ride in the bloodstream and like any normal human being the bloodstream goes everywhere and therefore there also goes the cancer seeking new organs to hit. It finds a weak cell structure and bingo it latches on and before you know it, it's metastatic. It doesn't stop there, it carries on and now of course, the blood is cancerous. Before long you have your scans and are told that the cancer is in so many places, now is the time to hit back. The only obvious way is Chemotherapy or Radiotherapy. Different treatments for different cancers. In my case for now it is Chemotherapy. There are of course various drug trials result in various types of Chemotherapy. As my cancer is a nasty, sneaky, aggressive one, they have hit me with 3 drugs, CISPLATIN, 5FU and

CISPLATIN with 5FU in a pump attached to me and going in 24/4. The cancer generally takes a hold. The only way is to hit it with treatments. Before long, the treatment then attacks the body cells including the cells that the cancer has latched on to. The cells that were just getting used to being hit by the Cancer now get hit by the treatment. The result is that the bad cells will die and also sometimes the Cancer in those actual cells. Good cells and mildly damaged cells will generally recover however and the same is repeated throughout the entire body. Eventually when the treatment can do no more it ends and the body may start to recover, if it can. Sometimes the treatment is so severe that the body may never recover and the Cancer may win. Having the Cancer can therefore be a double hit on the body and the body either dies from the cancer or the treatment or both. Some people go into remission and some do not. I have to be honest here, Cancer once it comes, rarely goes away. It gives the appearance of going away but in reality it just hides itself. It's a very devious disease. Many, many people have a good final result to treatment and live many years past their prognosis time limit. I am sorry if I have hurt you in any way with my writing. Believe you me, it is a living hell on earth and it will control your life for many many years. With Cancer you can never really plan ahead, if you do leave the next couple of years and then just pencil it in for two years time. That is how long is the average initial invasion time a cancer takes to enter and with treatment then stop having an effect on the body. Of course that is not the case to those poor people that are killed by cancer. The earlier you are diagnosed, the earlier you get treatment and fight back and then you have more of a chance to live longer. Cancer wants the easy quick way out and will try to kill you in a matter of months. In my case as you know, I am at stage 4 diagnosis with expected time to live of 18 months, my date that it will be all over for me is expected to be June 23rd 2015. Okay, I think I have said enough today on here. The anti-sickness is working so far and it's time now to take some more, take it easy and get some rest, maybe some sleep. Good Night all...

——— # # # ———

Good Morning All, FEBRUARY 27th 2014. Not a great day today. No sick during the night so my anti-sickness worked, then it all changed from around 6.30am this morning. What a transformation and change since yesterday evening and last night. I have been hanging over the toilet bowl and puking up with sweat, choking, crying and total bloody fatigue. Now it's time to expose the reality behind a mystery. Remember that smell that I got on several occasions, that smell I now know the full cause of it and what it is. The smell is obvious, new but so, so obvious now. When I do not flush the toilet after passing urine, the smell is a cocktail mix of the 3 drug Chemotherapy, urine and water all mixed together. When you think about it, the mix is already done inside my body before I expel by passing the urine into the toilet bowl. The surface of the water in the toilet bowl has the appearance of oil slick colours and stains in the water. It is all a mix combination of Chemotherapy chemicals reacting with urine. I apologise if this is a nasty description of that smell but I only want to show and tell you or to anyone what actually happens with simple urine passing. Now I have to add this to my list. It's no longer a secret or that elusive mystery. Nothing else to add today unless something exciting or interesting happens. I may actually sleep all day whether I go back to bed or just lay down. There is an actual example of having no plans and my life on hold while this is going on. I think that this may be the story of the coming days and nights where nearly every day is the same. So until we meet again very soon or … later, Cheerio.

——— # # # ———

GOOD MORNING again. Today is FRIDAY FEBRUARY 28th 2014 ... so Hello all. Today the usual. Up at 7am vomiting violently, violent sweaty, hurting pain, but there is something else. No it's not the smell from the chemo filled urine and not flushing. We've sussed that and it's on the list of bloody reactions to the treatment … Let me tell you! It's early days but this fatigue is taking a turn for the worse. During the morning between my vomiting expeditions. My expeditions are not Up Mount Everest, not Up The Amazon or The Nile and not to The North and South Poles. My expeditions are the trips to the vomiting zone in the toilet. Anyway, I went downstairs for a glass of cold water and each step took a bit of an effort. Now all these things happen at night. When I am resting or have had some sleep. I was slow on the steps going down but coming back up has shocked me. Yesterday and last night was okay. Things have changed! I had trouble coming back up those stairs, I was never an athlete on the stairs but it's totally different this morning, slower. I had to go very slowly and stop at every stop. I had to stop halfway to catch my breath and then carry on. At the stop I had to stop again. So 14 steps and I had to stop at step 7 and 14 and again at the top to get my breath back. It is getting worse and it's new and I bloody hate it. I hate it because it's different and I don't know how to handle it and no idea if it will get any worse and how do I cope with it. Is it the cancer in its new secondary place or is it Chemotherapy. I'm in limbo and I feel los. How bad will it get? If it affects my breathing, will I need to carry Oxygen around with me. Now my mind is playing tricks and I need to go back to bed and sleep. I am taking with me some fluids. Okay all, talk later or tomorrow. I thought I could write more but it got to me.. Sorry all! Cheerio xx

——— # # # ———

Good Morning all. It's SATURDAY MARCH 1sr 2014, and Happy Birthday to my Garreth (Gaz), my only child. A great son he is and I love him so much. He's a good boy and always was. It is Saturday morning and have a big red blotchy rash on neck and face. Maybe the medication is making it bad or part of the cause or maybe a reaction to treatment. Either way it's anti-sickness time in case I start vomiting or even feel nausea. I know now to leave taking my morning medication until after my morning puking up which is now almost guaranteed every morning. I can then take the medication and not puke it back up. For 3 days now, apart from Garreth and my sister, nobody else has called me. Even though Garreth is working full time he still calls me every day to keep an eye on me. Then he also pops by to stay now and then. I couldn't ask for anything more, could I now? As for me, it's time for a shower. Lucky I got one on the same level as the bedroom. That's the shower done. I went very slowly down the stairs and took on some fluids and fortisip which is a build up drink of 300 calories. My calorie intake is now very, very low because it tastes metallic and I still have a gastric band in place with near maximum restriction. My weight has dropped a bit. I think the only other option is to go back to bed. My body feels a little colder today. Right, am back in bed and that's where I am staying for the rest of today. I cannot see myself leaving this at all now for what's remaining of today. March 1st eh! St Davids Day and this David is staying in bed. Talk later, sorry write later I mean. Take care all. Oh before I go I still have not heard anything about my applications for PIP and ESA. It will mean extra money for me per week when my sick money comes to an end. My employers are already putting pressure on me. They have no care and never have done. I have seen what they are like in my 20 years working for them. They are ruthless people even though I have cancer and possibly dying a slow death. Good night all.

——— # # # ———

Hi all, it is SUNDAY MARCH 2ND 2014 and it's shower time. I think there's a good chance I am going to attend mass this morning at 10am. I will go to mass as often as I can but I realise that not being able to go will also happen some time. Okay gotta have this shower. Was vomiting earlier around 6.15am. It's now 8am so will write after it ... Hi all again, well I have had fun for the past 3 hours. No mass today for me. My vomiting has not stopped and it has been relentless non stop vomiting. It is draining me and it seems now that it is every day now For anybody reading this and not suffering from cancer even maybe not even knowing anyone with this cursed disease, then let me ask you something. First of all good for you if you haven't been touched by cancer, long may it continue, but tell me this, what is a normal thing for you in the morning or maybe towards the end of your normal daily sleep pattern. Well, whatever it is, how would you liken to be in my shoes or in the shoes of anyone suffering from Cancer and having large amounts of Chemotherapy or Radiotherapy. A normal morning for a cancer sufferer having Chemotherapy is the constant puking up. The main problem then with this is that this puking is without warning and my God it hurts and it's messy and it has no respect for the human body or the time of the day it happens. It is a by product of cancer. Cancer also tries to make friends with everyone. You don't know when it does this until it's too damn late. Getting rid of it is awful. You know we've all been there when you just can't shake off that "friend" that won't let go once they got a grip. Eventually you do get rid but the anguish, pain and personal private loneliness is a living nightmare.

Everyone has experienced a sleepless night from time to time but with cancer, it rarely goes while the mind is on constant overdrive working out how, why and what if? etc. A normal morning or day for most people is work or leisure activities, shopping, school, college, the Gym or travel. To me and any normal cancer treatment recipient a normal morning or day is getting used to various normal treatment reactions. At the moment I am at the treatment stage reaction mainly in the mornings with my head stuck in a toilet bowl. The view is not great while the contents of my stomach are emptied into that toilet bowl. It's gruesome and graphic but I have to clearly explain what I am going through and what a person about to receive treatment will probably face depending on the amount of Chemotherapy facing soon or planned by your consultant.... As the vomit is dragged from the pit of your stomach on the way up and eventually out, it leaves your mouth and hits the sides of the bowl or whatever you are using. Sometimes you may be unlucky not to make the toilet in time. Anyhow for me as it hits the bowl sides, it then hits the water in the toilet. The inevitable happens and some of it splashes back up and hits you in the face. There is nothing to hate, it's your own vomit. Then the smell hits you, the smell of vomit reacting with urine because I forgot to flush the toilet earlier and of course there is that other smell of chemo mixed with urine. The toilet was not flushed because you had no idea when this vomiting would actually begin. None of this is pleasant at all, is it? but it isn't stopping. Fifteen minutes in and I am still emptying any thing in my stomach into that bowl. That bowl by now is the only friend I have ... The phone rings and guess what, I cannot detach myself from this bowl and the actual vomiting. Also I cannot forget the vomit splashes on my face and without a mirror could be in other places as well. I touch my face and it is wet, very wet from vomit and now sweat. I am exhausted and the sweat is pouring out of me. My body is now in shock and now the shortness of breath makes itself known to me. Thirty minutes have now gone and cramp is appearing in both my legs and stomach. I cannot move and eventually after 40 to 45 minutes it all stops as there is nothing left in my stomach to come out. I fall back down on the floor totally wiped out from what has just happened over the best part of the last hour. I then cried and screamed for help from anywhere. I cried and cried and cried. I cried because there was nothing left in me to come out but tears. Vomiting was over for now. My crying and screaming was in fear of me not being able to get up off the floor. I had no idea what was going to happen next and yet I should know because this is exactly what happens most days or evenings now. It is a scary dark place to be alone on the floor, covered in splashed vomit, sweating, violent headaches and to think that all I want is to be healthy again but then again, my consultant Theresa says that I am going to eventually be killed by this f*****g Cancer. I feel depressed and more lonely but I can also feel my strength coming into my legs as I struggle and eventually get up, close the toilet bowl lid and wipe my tears away and think to myself, what has happened. But I know, I know what happened, I know why. I go through it most days This is my average routine on most mornings and sometimes afternoons depending on what happens overnight as my treatment progresses and if I am forced to remain in bed for rest. As you can see it is 40 minutes or so that takes a toll on my body. Of course the recovery then takes so much longer to get to a level where I can then try to attempt to cope with whatever hits me next. As the Chemotherapy levels build up in my body, then this 45 minutes can only get longer and very, very difficult even to the point of almost being unbearable.

I have been allocated as treatment, three large Chemotherapy drugs of CISPLATIN, 5FU and CETUXIMAB and also the pump doing its work 24/4 rather than 24/7. On top of that 45 minute routine which is the daily worst there are of course other puking incidents during the day which are shorter sequences of various lengths of time but still consisting of the vomiting, sweating and equalling exhausting results. Some of these other sessions are also lasting sometimes as long and with equal energy wasting. As I have many weeks to go yet, you can appreciate why my condition will deteriorate further as the treatment progresses. All of these sessions of violent vomiting hit me every time with absolutely violent headaches, scary headaches. So you are very lucky if you are doing anything other than morning, daily, even hourly episodes of violent, sweaty vomiting. You get the picture, it is not nice, never has been and never will be. It's evening now and it has been a truly debilitating day but I had to show and explain what I go through now every single day as my cancer continues to get hit by Chemotherapy treatment and to think it is all to just hope that I can buy extra time to live. For tonight shall I say Goodnight. Tomorrow I shall so to speak "pick up my pen again" and continue to show everyone what my cancer and treatment is doing to me. Sleeping, crying, sweating and vomiting has been my day today. Tomorrow is another day, GOODNIGHT ALL.

——— # # # ———

Good Morning All IT IS MONDAY MARCH 3rd 2014, had a cup of tea at 8am this morning and as yet still hasn't come up. What I mean is that I havent got sick yet. Give it time, vomiting in my case needs no encouragement. It's Monday and the start of a new week. Being a Monday also means one more thing, yes, it's Chemo all inclusive Infusion day and as we know by now the reason I call it that is because I get a lovely wristband with all my details on it to identify me and in return I get all their lovely Chemotherapy chemicals. I know by now off by heart my Hospital number 5*3**4*T .... I will never forget that number as long as I live and just in case anyone thinks I have, no, I have not based any of my lottery numbers on it. That may change if I go into remission but highly unlikely as my condition is terminal. Today is one Chemo Drug Cetuximab day so it's at least 3 hours in Guys. The needlework for that starts at 1.30pm. It is now 9.45am and time to get motivated for it all, back later ...

Hi there again ... it's 11.30am and as luck would have it I have just been hugging my mate which is the toilet bowl for the last 35 minutes. As you now that's not too bad for me, a short one. Still had the usual connected sweats and cramps. My rash is also very bad this morning and now under my right eye is a new thing where the skin is also getting dry and flaky and hence very embarrassing. I have booked a cab from Cannon Cars for 12 noon. I don't really mind if I get to Guys early as long as I get there. As you know I pass the time there watching the world go by and I listen to the others around me. It's a laugh just listening to other people deciding on other peoples afflictions just by looking at them. These people who criticize other people around them are themselves the most hideous forms of human beings themselves, but I look, learn and am amused by them. This is what makes the world go by and it passes the time and I sometimes wonder what did some people decide for me last week and if it has changed this week. Human nature is very humorous. Anyhow, I done my cab trip and train trip to London Bridge. One thing I did notice today is that my walk from the Station in London Bridge to Guys was more tiring than the last time and the short distance took me longer than before. Now is when I notice those little things happening more and more that are taking more of a toll on my body. I had felt queasy leaving the house and even though I had my extra 35 minutes earlier vomiting the life out of me, I have a strange feeling it's going to happen again despite having taken the anti-sickness medication earlier as I left the house to go to the station in Orpington. I now carry a black rucksack everywhere I go. In it is a phone charger, charging power pack, water, 2 days supply of all my medication, full bottle of anti-sickness medication, tissues and of course my mobile phone. At home my next job will be to prepare a bag in case I am taken to hospital without warning. Anyhow the usual has happened as regards my chemotherapy infusion. It took 3 hours and apart from when Gaz came to see me, I slept through most of it. We all know that cancer disregards all ages, colour, creeds and sex. It just does not care and even though I have been attending here now since January 2nd I thought I saw it all until today.

I met a young man, a father of 3 kids and his young wife. He is 27 years old, kids are 5, 3 and just under 2 years old. His wife is just aged 28. The sad thing is that he is just like me he too has been diagnosed with Head and Neck Cancer a tumour in the back of his throat and it's metastatic. His prognosis is also like mine at 18 months maximum to live. Alex is his name and his wife is Karen. Karen at 28 and with 3 young kids has her work cut out, a mortgage and a sick possibly dying husband/dad. The eldest at 5 realises his dad is very, very sick. The 3 year old boy and the younger little girl of course do not realise the full story of their dad. To them dad is dad who is sick and that's it. Karen is very tearful and has absolutely no idea what she is going to do. She has a strong family support and my God she is going to need it. If the worst happens, what are those kids going to do without a dad. Alex like me is in the early stages of treatment and of course is more worried about his wife and kids than himself. We chatted a lot and will look out for each other as our treatment progresses on our similar journey with this cancer. Of course our treatment days and times may be different but our end intention is the same, yes, both of us will try to beat the 18 months prognosis. Anyhow, also around me today were 2 patients with what I call "jockey helmets", you know the ones with the cold water to save hair loss during chemotherapy. Women are the most likely wearers of this headgear. As regards all the nurses names, I still do not know all of them. Of the staff and nurses, I know only Lucy, Aoife, Catherine, Lauren, Jennifer, Stephen, Gary, Meeta, Alison. Then the staff Richard, Evelyn and Heena. Today my nurse Alison is from Manchester. These nurses certainly put in long shifts, long days and their devotion to this Chemotherapy treatment is certainly admirable. I am in awe of what they do. Also today I forgot to tell you that I was called for a blood test and I was seen reasonably on time. My 1.30pm appointment and I was in Cubicle 1 in Zone C. Gaz came to me at 2pm as usual. After my one drug Cetuximab infusion session, I was on a train home after 5pm. It was busy and even though it was cold and packed, I just wanted to get home. I was tired and now with less energy to fight for a seat. No vomiting either so maybe the anti-sickness is working, or maybe it's just today and the huge sessions of vomiting will come to me at home.

As soon as I got home, the energy just departed my body so quickly. I have steps up to both my front door and rear door. I was heading in the back entrance to my kitchen and I just could not get the energy to lift my legs and get up those back steps to the door. I struggled and eventually got there. I had to catch my breath. I reached up to the top shelf and got a tin of oxtail soup. It was then I realised that it would taste like metal or paper but I had to get some calories into me. Then something else hit me. I was facing those steps upstairs as I had to get to the loo. Yes it was smelly urine discharge time. I left the soup and began the long climb. After two stops I had to stop and rest for at least a minute. Another 2 and rest. Another 3 stops and I was totally wiped out. A similar amount of steps remained so after a few minutes I did the remaining individually by moving, stopping, moving and stopping. In all, the stairs had taken me over 20 minutes. Yesterday was absolutely nothing like this, My God what a deteriorating state my health has become in a day. What am I going to do? My single Chemo infusion days of Cetuximab like today take up over 3 hours also in Guys as well as travelling to and from the Cancer Day Unit, when put together near 6 hours. When I have a day of 3 chemo drugs and taking into account the travelling it takes up to 10 or 11 hours away from home morning to evening. I dread the future as my body continues to get worse, it scares me what may lie ahead. I think today is probably my 10th day of chemotherapy and it is only near halfway. What the hell will I be like next week not to mention in another 10 or 11 weeks. Each day now I see myself getting worse. Also every day Gaz calls me and we chat. It is so, so nice. Gaz, my only child, should not be in this position watching his dad go through this hell, it's also hell for him to go through this. I feel so, so lucky to have Gaz with me and then I have the added bonus of him coming to see me in Guys during treatment day on the 10th floor. He has been on my journey with me. My God I remember it now and think of it every day when he learned of my bad news. I am lucky to have him. He is so strong. He lost his mum in 2008, I will do all I can that he doesn't lose me too early. Bless you Garreth, you continue to do me so proud. He never lets me down. In 2008 he was a fresher in Durham University when my wife Joan (his mum) took ill suddenly. I got him back home only hours before she passed away in Intensive Care at The Princess Royal University Hospital. After the funeral in New Year 2009, Garreth went back to Durham University for the 3 year course in Computer Science and done his mum and me so proud by graduating with a 2:1 in Computer Science. He is now an IT Business Consultant and continues to do so well in life. I am both proud and delighted for you Garreth. You shouldnt have to go through all this shit with me but life is the toss of a coin. Again thanks Gaz and I love you so much and always will. That is it for today, Good night all.

——— # # # ———

GOOD MORNING ALL. It's TUESDAY MARCH 4th 2014. After I had gone to bed so early, it's now 4am and am up vomiting and sweating. Got it all out of the way, yes the magic twosome, vomit and sweat. It lasted 5 or 6 minutes and now am going back to bed. I also just realised that my energy is gone, slow on my feet but not missed the toilet bowl yet ... Okay back to bed … Hi, am up for a vomit and to pass urine, yes a puke and a pee. I hugged the bowl but not for too long. My energy levels are gone however I was told that the day would come when I would not leave my sick bed, so in the meantime I will get up if I can, get sick, get showered or washed, get dressed and get the hell downstairs. The trick is to do it as early as possible … Hi again, yes I got downstairs for 12 noon and just watched TV. My rash is itchy now with some flaky skin. I am tired, very tired and actually want to sleep all the time. I keep thinking how fast I have gone downhill as it is only been a matter of weeks. I suppose that is what massive amounts of chemotherapy does to the human body, my body. To sum up today, bad rash, flaky skin, tired, sweating and vomiting. I have no more today. Sorry too tired to write to the diary now. Again I am sorry, maybe write later if I get energy to do so … Okay, Hi all again. Because my energy levels are getting very erratic, there may now be some days that nothing will happen or that I am too exhausted to write. As regards this book, I will hold nothing back and will write as much as I legally can and if it happens to me, then it will be entered into this writing that I am doing. I also have many photos and some are bad and graphic so far and I have no doubt the others to follow will be similar. All photos at a later date will be published also. My reason is that I expect there will be physical changes to my body. So as of today now it is 8.30am and now I have a pain in my throat. As the days go by, things are quite simply getting bloody awful as the days go by. I haven't heard yet about my upcoming appointment to see Theresa, my consultant, but it will be soon though as Theresa does like to keep tabs on me and also I trust her to give me the correct treatment and buy me some extra time. As I have already said, I have trusted Dr Theresa Guerrero-Urbano since I was diagnosed. I also believe she will do her best to buy me some extra time to live. She knows what is best and in effect my life is in her hands. For the rest of today I am going to take it easy, maybe if I feel better later I could pop out to do some shopping. I need to get ginger nut biscuits. I have been told that they are a different taste when all I can taste at the moment is metallic or paper from my food. I have not eaten today at all and as it is getting late now there won't be any food for me to take today. I will start losing weight soon enough then the hospital will require me to take in build up drinks to keep energy as good as possible. Anyhow unless anything else happens, I will sign out and write again tomorrow….

——— # # # ———

GOOD DAY TO YOU ALL. It is WEDNESDAY MARCH 5th 2014, and so far today, no vomiting as yet, but that could happen at any time, a red itchy flaky rash in my face and neck. Now it's so dry and flaky it resembles dandruff and falls about everywhere. I am tired, no energy, sweating a lot and crying a lot. The crying is bad because it happens without warning and if it happens while shopping, I just stop and then people look at me like I am a crazy man. People are so quick to judge when it comes to seeing anybody cry in public and in my case a man crying is the ultimate for them. I also sweat so much, again a part of the sickness even in cold weather. But as yet, no sick today up to now. I am very tired with sod all energy. it doesn't help that I have not eaten. However I am very lonely and feel depressed, crying and thinking. All these f*****g people saying that they are here for me, well I'm beginning to weed them out. Fakes is what they are, fake people with their fake families even fakes in my family. In life they have loved themselves but failed me. It wouldn't be too much trouble if I died now. They might go to the funeral, but only to make their appearance and to be seen. As time goes by, I will surely find the others. The longer I live the more of them I expose. God it's terrible when I discover that there are fakes in my own family, as I said before not immediate family. These distant fake family people are those that I have never spoken to and I will never speak or contact them for as long as I live. Forgive me for appearing to go on and on about fakes but they have shocked me by their actions. Everybody has fakes in their family, it's just a small matter of trying to find them. Don't look too hard, the fakes always show their true colours when they look for attention. The fakes in my family are distant relations. Let me give you an example. I have very distant family members yet since I got sick they have never once enquired about me and I can guarantee you they will stay in their own little world and couldn't care f*****g less if I ever existed. I then have close family members at the moment who cannot accept the fact that I have cancer. My own very close immediate family bless him, I love him dearly and at first he was slow to contact me, but no, sadly he simply cannot accept the fact that I have cancer. I don't really mind as some people are different accepting shit things burdened by their family. I hope one day that the situation changes and I think it will. I do not want to die before he realises and accepts the fact that I have cancer. He may have only 18 months or less to change and realise the situation. I say to everyone out there reading this, do not wait to say nice things at your family member's funeral, and the same to people who know me, come and visit me now and say the nice things. If I die before this book is published then that last message is falling on deaf ears. I am currently drawing up a list of all those that have failed me and continue to fail me and also those who will shortly fail me, believe me I know who you are and by what you are doing now to me, I know you will fail me. Fake family and fake friends. Everybody knows who they are and the sad thing is that every family has them. Sometimes the fakes themselves do not realise that they are ass holes ... OKAY. I will write again later or tomorrow. xxx

——— # # # ———

MARCH 6th. 2014 THURSDAY. Overnight has been hell violent vomiting, rash pain everywhere, no energy, very weak. YES, I am bad and if it continues I may call an ambulance. I am very bad, sorry for this but it is going to be a day of bed and toilet, violent vomiting, sweating, feeling low and I am alone. Thank you, Let me try to write again tomorrow. CHEERIO EVERYONE.

——— # # # ———

GOOD MORNING everybody, it is FRIDAY MARCH 7th 2014. Another day, another repeat of downright sickness, depression, loneliness, no eating, drinking water yes, but yes to more vomiting, sick in head and body, tiredness, weak no energy, very bad flaky red rash and generally BAD. I say bad but every day is bad now and every day seems a little worse than the previous day. I find myself doing a lot of thinking, stupid thinking and it does nothing for me. I cry a lot just like when I lost my Joan back in 2008. Never saw it coming, and after that I cried for no bloody reason whatsoever. Maybe now it's because I am lonely and I have cancer, here we go again, alone. What scares me most is dying alone. I don't want to die, who does?, but I do not want to die alone. Although with cancer the chances are high that I will die with a nurse by my side in a hospital or a hospice. I don't really care as long as I do not die alone. At the moment the only way I could die alone is if it was by my own hand, but yes, I can't believe I wrote this but here it is in my diary. For the past couple of weeks I have thoughts about suicide in one form or another. I feel now that the only person who loves me is Garreth my son, my only child. If I didn't have Garreth I think I would be gone by now. Without Gaz, I have absolutely no reason to stay alive. I am not leaving Garreth on his own. Bless you and Thank you Garreth. Yes, I have family in Ireland but that's in Ireland, not here right beside me. I could quite easily take the paracetamol way out but I have Gaz. I can tell you now that if you or anybody is in a similar position with all the reactions to your cancer and treatment doing stupid things to your mind and body, then be prepared to also be thinking of doing yourself in at one stage or another. Dealing with cancer is something you certainly cannot do on your own. So, If you are just beginning to deal with having Cancer and you are on your own, please get someone you know or trust or dependable to be with you right from the beginning. I promise you, you cannot do it on your own. If you chose to go it alone, you will definitely not complete the journey in full. If you are on your own, you will fall by the wayside and you will not get up. Trust me, it is absolute hell. I am stopping writing now. I do not want to feel any more depressed than this tomorrow. Take care all. Tomorrow is another day.

——— # # # ———

Hi all. It is SATURDAY MARCH 8th 2014. The usual applies to me today, tired, bad itchy rash, no energy, vomiting, stomach pains, crying, sweating and depression feelings. What can I say, I get all the above and it is hurtful. Deep down from the pit of my stomach and the deepest part of my heart I am in absolute pure hell. I hate myself and I don't know what I'm going to do when things get worse. You might say the same as some people when they say "OH DON'T WORRY"or "IT'LL BE ALL RIGHT"or "YOU'LL BE OKAY", well it's not the case, it couldn't be. I got Cancer, there is nothing worse in life other than losing someone close. the next worse thing in life is getting cancer. It is Saturday and I've decided to take things easy. No more today, I will write again tomorrow...

——— # # # ———

GOOD MORNING, IT'S SUNDAY MARCH 9th 2014, tiredness, bad red itchy flaky rash, vomiting, sweating, no energy getting around and intense feelings of loneliness. I'm going to mass today as tomorrow is Monday and am facing a 3 drug infusion day in Guys Hospital, 10th floor, my second home, but back to today and now I just got a random feeling that I need to cry. First is Mass and maybe cry when it does happen. I have to go to mass when I can because it will happen that I cannot go. Mass is at 10am and it's now 8.30am. one and a half hours from now and when I get home from mass about 12 noon, I will then write ...

HI THERE, not quite 12 noon, it's bloody 3pm and I feel depressed again. Mass didn't do a lot for me today. I probably went there hoping for a change in how I feel inside me. It didn't happen, all I got was the usual gossip merchants, The whispering people, the soft spoken and the nosey f*****s. As I said before, I love my catholic religion and my beliefs but as some people in my church are loving caring people, there are also so many that want to listen and then gossip. Then if the story is not what they expected, they make it up. Anyhow home now and as I give into this treatment the time is coming now where I may not be able to get to mass on Sunday morning at 10am in St Swithun's, Fashoda Road, Bromley, Kent.... I am home now and the tiredness is just shit. I have again puked up and as I knelt on the floor emptying my stomach into that toilet bowl, I can also feel the life and energy within me also disappearing down that same toilet bowl. I eventually stopped vomiting and then I had to plan my next move. To get up to a standing position from where I am on the floor is going to take a lot of energy to do it and then after doing it, I'm going to have to plan on trying to get downstairs. I did get up from the toilet floor and eventually after a little rest managed to get down the stairs. I know as I step by step slowly edged my footwork down each stair that as soon as I done 7 steps I had to stop. I stopped on the 7th step because I knew I had to stop and had a little rest. My God, I have really got worse even since yesterday. As I sat on that 7th step, I started to feel the tears well up in my eyes and I started to cry. I am suddenly totally devastated, wiped out mentally and physically. I am also more devastated by the fact that I have bloody cancer and I am not getting any better. Gaz and I speak of course every day, but he is busy with his job and I would not want that to change in any way. Mary my sister calls or texts me every day. It's all great, but I am f*****g dying. I know the chemotherapy forces me to be very sick in mind and body, medically and physically. Yes, Yes I know all that but right now I cannot comprehend all that. All I know is that I vomit regularly with little or no warning and another thing I know is that I am still in the middle of the stairs on the 7th step looking downwards at the remaining steps and the bottom of the stairs below me. Like my disease, I feel lost and lonely and I also know that I am still too tired to complete the rest of the way down the stairs to the bottom. I also know that I will then again have to rest on that last step just to get enough energy in me to get to the sofa in my front room. Good God I may even decide to go back up, rest half way up and again at the top step and go to bed. Such is the state of my condition right now. I just haven't got the energy to make a simple decision right now. How long will I be here. Right now my whole life is happening on the 7th step of my stairs. I hope I am not beginning to sound boring but that's what it is right now. I will be here for as long as it takes on Step 7 of my stairs. I looked at my watch and it's only 3.10pm in the afternoon or near it …

Hi again... It's only been 10 or 12 minutes, yes it's 3.25 pm and I'm on the move. I am going down, but I know now that I will have to allow 30 to 45 minutes to go back up those stairs to bed. That has been the longest it has taken to go downstairs so again the once previous gradual decline of my body and its condition is changing. I now feel that the downhill progression of my whole body is really speeding up. How long is it now? I think this is about the 10th week into the 18 week treatment plan. Is it any wonder that things are bad. Every time I have the 3 drug chemotherapy session like what I am facing tomorrow, I used to gradually recover after a week even though I had it pumping into me as well over another 4 days before the district nurse disconnection. Then it is yes for it in time for the 1 drug session a week later and then again for the following week session one drug infusion. That is such a lot of Chemotherapy that the once slight recovery afterwards will possibly very soon maybe this week or next week come to an end and I will not know the difference from one week to the next. My mental state will get far worse. I will again think about death by my own doing but I also want to live and not leave Garreth on his own. He is there for me and I am going to be there for him. Today, I have also noticed extra things happening to me. My hair on my head is feeling brittle and soft. My facial hair is beginning not to need shaving. The hair on my head was always cut tight anyway. Now my hair is in limbo, it's not falling out and it's not growing. My toenails and fingernails too are feeling strange but I cannot put my finger on the problem yet. I am also noticing pins and needles and tingling feelings in my fingertips and toes. Again this is all new to me but I'm sure this cancer and chemotherapy has many more tricks up its sleeve. I will write again once I've negotiated the big stair climb journey to bed later.... Well I made it to bed.... It was like the planning and implementation of an epic adventure matching any adventure movie but to me it was just about leaving my front room, getting fluids on board, heading for those 14 steps of the stairs climbing them in stages and after using the toilet got undressed, then it's into bed. In the bedroom before getting into bed, I had to make sure that there was a clear uninterrupted pathway to the loo. If I was going to get a bout of vomiting which was very, very likely, and knowing my slow footwork would more than likely be a shuffle rather than a dash to the toilet bowl but I still had to make sure that the route to it was clear. Anyhow I am going to sleep and I hope for a good night sleep with little interruptions. Good night all, and I will write again in the morning. Bless you all.

——— # # # ———

MORNING ALL IT'S MONDAY March 10th 2014. I had a reasonable night but the sick sweaty puking up happened at 6am and on and off lasted until 7.45am. In all that time I never left the toilet bowl once. As before, I was hanging over the toilet bowl emptying my guts into it and while vomiting, I could feel the life inside me also flowing out of me with the vomit into the bowl. I was sweating so much that on two occasions. I barely got a few feet away from that bowl when I felt sick again. Once was enough to be surprised by more vomiting but twice knocked the shit out of me. For 1 hour and 45 minutes my whole life was into this toilet bowl and little space around it. When I eventually finished the only liquid in me was the actual sweat pumping out of me. It's hell without a rest. I have to recover now and get ready for my Chemotherapy later in Guys at 12 noon for my All Inclusive Chemo day. Six hours plus in the Cancer Day Unit as well as a possible earlier blood test beforehand and then the struggle home with that usual pump attached for the next four days. Because of that random blood test, I am going to leave here early if I can and then my Chemo will not be delayed too much as it has before because of a delayed blood test result. If I go in around 9.30am, should get there around 10.15am to the main entrance and take it from there. My train with off peak charges on my Oyster Card was after 9.30am. As I got off the train in London Bridge, I felt exhausted. The quick-paced morning had caught up with me and now I had no choice but to hold up the pace and go slowly down the slope from the platform at London Bridge down the tunnel and down the escalator, through the barrier, turn left and follow the wall right to the end past the flower stall and the Jehovah's Witnesses. I walked over the pedestrian crossing and past MacDonalds. Then at the left past the Sainsburys local that does the hospital prescriptions and then finally along to the Guys Hospital entrance, through the revolving doors and into the Hospital foyer and all that went on. It was all a struggle today more so than last week. I literally had to shuffle all the way to Guys Hospital. Inside my body was ice cold yet to keep warm I had a black puffer jacket zipped up with a hood on my head. Inside that I had a heavy jumper, black scarf, gloves and a wool hat. To look at me I did resemble a typical cancer patient undergoing chemotherapy. I was pale, tired, sweaty yet ice cold, feeling sick or nausea and feeling pain. It was not big pain but that lingering annoying pain. I did not want to be where I am right now. To be truthful, I actually did not want to be alive, but alive I am and I have a little fight in me that tops the decision balance towards wanting to be alive for another twenty four hours or even a week. Right now, I just want to live through today long enough to have treatment and wake up sometime tomorrow hopefully feeling the same. I don't know if I will feel like that or not. However today is massive Chemo for over 6 hours infusion plus a chemo pump going home. I have to do it or I will die. I decided to go straight to the 10th floor Cancer Day Unit. I did the usual, handed over my blue appointment card and in return I got my All Inclusive white wristband. I was told that I had to undergo a blood test before treatment. If blood was okay then chemo would go ahead. It was a struggle to get here, and I got here ahead of time to allow for this no warning blood test. I do not want any cancellations now at this late stage. My name was called and off I went into the side room for this blood test. All over in a few minutes and went back outside and took my seat in the waiting room again. I still felt cold and kept my hat on. A nurse appeared and called a name, not mine. I looked around politely smiled and nodded. Around me were some really sick looking people, hairless heads and looking pale and sick. Today I now looked exactly like one of them around me so I blended in. It's strange but as I now looked like this, I justified my reason for being here. I was a terminal cancer patient and I was now undergoing treatment. Today I can clearly see around me 9 people looking very sick and two looking reasonably healthy. I got it right, bang on, no mistakes today, all of the nine were cancer patients well into their treatment and the other two were a carer and a family member.

One thing that I must remember is that looking reasonably better after treatment by Chemotherapy does not begin until near enough 7 to 9 weeks after treatment actually ends. Going by that and today is March 10th, and that I have a lot of treatment and recovery to do yet, If I am to get through it, I will not look any better until into next year 2015. Can you imagine, the rest of my year is now definitely to be cancelled, wiped out. God I dread the future even more now. Just before 12.30pm I was called by Claire one of the Cancer Day Unit nurses. Claire is from Manchester. She took me to Zone C and Cubicle 10. I was sharing the cubicle with 3 other patients who are already connected up to their infusion machines and the chemical cocktail of various Chemotherapy is already flowing into their bodies. I took my lounger, sat in it and waited for it all to begin. Checking my wristband, verifying my identity was what Claire and another nurse did next, the treatment began first with getting fluid into me, This was followed by the Piriton which eventually would make me sleep. Garreth (Gaz) came to visit me on his lunch break. It is always nice to see him and after he left to go back to work the treatment just carried on. The clear liquid bags of chemicals are lined up for infusion into me. As you know they are CISPLATIN, 5FU and CETUXIMAB and going home with a pump of 5FU. The pump is what I don't like but gotta put up with it for now. My stay here today will be for over 6 hours. Anyhow, now that the treatment is established here for today and Garreth is gone back to work, I think it's time for me to sleep. I know I won't be leaving here until 6.30pm or 7pm tonight. At least that time the train will be easy to get a seat on my way home. For now it's sleep time. Before that a nurse came up to me and said that my rash was now very noticeable and a doctor was on the way to see it and prescribe something for it. It was now 4pm and for a nurse to comment on it, then it must be getting bad and obvious. Just as I drifted off to sleep a doctor appeared and prescribed a cream that I would get in Sainsburys Chemist later. As treatment continued, I drifted off to sleep as I always do. At around 6.30pm, I woke again and two nurses were doing the closing treatments and flushing out my PICC Line. After having the pump connected, I should be out of here in 15 minutes. I left at 6.55pm and had to go to the Pharmacy on the way to the Station. I collected from there some Aveeno Cream and Doxycycline capsules. It took me a while to get out of there and I shuffled to London Bridge Station. This trip to the Pharmacy and the wait took up a lot of time. I got to the Station just before 8pm. Took the train to Orpington and taxi home. I got home indoors at 9.15 pm. I took fluids on board and slowly in stages climbed the stairs to bed. I was in bed by 10.10pm and crashed out. This bloody pump is very awkward though. I briefly woke to go to the loo at 11.50pm. Then I had to rest on the loo, I was wiped out and got back to bed just before 1am. Okay so it's bloody Tuesday morning 11th March but I need my sleep. No vomiting so far or should I say, yet. Trust me it will happen. I haven't done a day without vomiting yet and today will be no exception.

——— # # # ———

TUESDAY MARCH 11th 2014. GOOD MORNING ALL. Do you know but today I feel different, yes I was only a little sick in the early hours of the morning. I was up at 11.50pm and got back to bed at 1am. It was a smelly wee. As you know, detecting that smell took weeks and weeks but it was the damn chemicals in my urine all along. Same story this morning for me and now every time I go to pass urine, I get that smell that I will never forget and another thing I noticed is that when I now pass urine, I look down at the water in the toilet bowl and I see my reflection and something else new, different colours in the water like petrol or diesel or oil mixing in the water and causing these colours in the water. Very strange what these chemicals do to me or anybody having them pumped into them. Also at this time I got sick again but only a little. Anyhow it's 10am and I have to have a shower. God knows it's gonna take me a long time to get that out of the way but no matter how sick I get, I am determined to wash every day in some way or another. If nothing else, I need to keep clean. I should be able to write later to you all. Well can you believe it, two hours ago sickness and vomiting paid me a visit and it's just finished. It is now just before 1pm. Not a lot to do for the rest of today. I'm going to stay out of bed now for as long as possible today unless I have no choice in the matter. I struggled to get downstairs, step-by-step, short rest at step 8 today and on getting to the bottom, I stopped and rested on that bottom step. While catching my breath, I realised that today I had to get to the chemist. I have called them earlier as up to now my cancer treatment connected medication was coming from Guys and the chemist near my doctors was delivering it to me.

Today is a little different as I have to collect boxes of Fortisip build up drinks. Each flavoured bottle is 300 calories and is a quick easy way to maintain my weight and put a stop to any weight loss getting worse. Weight loss is a problem lately and this should put a stop to this. Most of my food and drink tastes like metal or paper. I hope that these drinks are swift and effective. Eventually I got to the chemist by driving. Driving is no problem for me and it's actually nice to get out. I picked up two big boxes of FORTISIP drinks and got them home. When I got home, I opened my back gate and garage and put the car away safe and secure out of the way. I knew that I did not want to go anywhere for the rest of the week. Once the car was parked in the garage, I realised that my body could not move even the slightest. I rested up but had no idea then that I was wiped out and I had no option but to stay in that drivers seat for 35 to 40 minutes. From now on I have to be careful in case it happens again when I am not prepared for it. It was after 5pm and I listened to LBC on the car radio. This now also tells me that I must now buy myself a walking stick to help me get around easier. Eventually at about 6pm, I had enough energy to leave the car and get indoors. It was dark and I shuffled up those few rear door steps into my home through the garden. After carefully doing those last few steps, I entered the kitchen and switched on the kettle. I grabbed a chair and had to sit down. The short walk from the garage to the house was about 70 to 80 feet and had wiped me out. Twice I flicked that kettle on to re boil it and I eventually had a cuppa tea and a Fortisip drink. Fortisip is such a quick way to get calories into me. I secured the house and switched off all lights. At 9pm I slowly climbed the stairs to bed but also by doing my pit stops in between. The journey was a struggle but eventually I completed it. By 9.40pm I had gone to the loo and was tucked up in bed awaiting my night of vomiting ahead. For some strange reason I realised that my heating and radiators had been up full night and day 24/7 ever since I was diagnosed back in late 2013. That was going to be a nasty gas bill. Despite this I still felt ice cold inside. Anyhow, I got into bed as I said, switched on my radio and must have drifted off to sleep. Yes radio, I listen a lot to LBC Radio or Classic FM. I have listened to them for many years now. My favourite presenters on LBC are Nick Ferarri and James O Brien. I also take the time to listen to Katie Hopkins on whatever station she is in. She don't give a shit and she don't take shit. I love her view on life. Back to LBC and Nick Ferarri is on early morning followed at 10am by James O Brien. I love James and his mystery hour every Thursday at 12 noon until 1pm. I drift off to sleep with Classic FM. Tonight is Classic FM easy listening. Finally by 11.30pm I was drifting off to sleep and nothing was going to wake me apart from getting up to have a vomiting session, which as is very likely to happen. GOOD NIGHT ONE AND ALL.

——— # # # ———

GOOD MORNING. It's Wednesday March 12th 2014. Hurray. It's already the middle of the week but no vomiting today yet even though it's only 5.30am. It's cold but my radiators are on full. Makes no difference to me at all, night and day I feel the cold an awful lot now. Thermostat downstairs is 25°C and I am still freezing cold. I must remember to get onto MacMillan about my gas and electric bill. Another thing I notice is this pump has the 5FU Chemo drug in it, well this pump is getting on my tits, literally. I wear it and its straps draped across my shoulder right to left. The tube is going into my left upperarm 24/7 for 4 days. Now I find it difficult to have a shower while wearing it. It's possible to do it but it now takes forever as I get more and more tired. Still, on Friday night a district nurse must come out and disconnect and flush it out. Anyhow now time to have a shower, which is going to take ages. Another thing I notice today is a soreness in some toes. I think it's time to make an appointment with a chiropodist.

My God having cancer does take forever because of the many reactions to it and the treatments within the body. So many things are already happening to my body now. A lot of these I was not told anything about because now they are in a few months time. So many, many things happening to my body now. Like I said before, the incidents happen and the list then branches out from these incidents to create branches with other reactions and so on and so on. By the time I am well into treatment in a few months from now there may be hundreds of reactions in my body. However, now I reckon that the soreness in my toes is because of ingrowing toe nails. In some cases the Chemo stops hair growing and it may even fall out. Cases vary and as you know in my case, hair stops growing but in some parts grows out of control. Basically nails are like hair and in my case toe nails are growing out of control and are growing inwards. This is definitely what is happening to me right now and it will get worse, far worse and I have a long way to go yet. Chemo and Radiotherapy effects on the body carry on for many, many weeks after the actual treatment finishes. I really do not care as long as I do show some form of recovery in the end as that means for me, it will be next year before any recovery may start to show. Every day now seems to show an horrible reaction to my Chemotherapy. Nothing surprises me anymore, nothing does at all now, as that is why I kept an exact true to life, in depth diary entry of every single incident of every single day. Some days as my treatment progresses will show nothing happening and that is why my diary entries reflect any incidents. If nothing happens, nothing will be entered and there will be days like that like there will be days that everything goes mad. I am not creating any false stories. If it happened, then it is here. However I cannot name people unless they have given me permission to do so. It is crazy because one minute nothing happens maybe for hours on end and then mayhem when a new reaction happens. Believe me, it's the easiest thing in the world to give up and not take anymore. Look at me, I am having a day like that today now and has been like this for past few days ... Please, please, please put up with it if you can. It is far, far worse when you are feeling alone. The days and nights are shit, awful, sometimes unbearable, but remember one thing, IF YOU GIVE UP, YOU WILL SURELY DIE, (this is guaranteed), TAKE THE TREATMENT THEY OFFER YOU AND YOU JUST MAY LIVE. They know best so accept all help, not everybody is offered the treatment, Fight it and put up with the crap, the pains, the sweating, sore toes and ingrowing toenails and vomiting with pain. Remember one thing, it is a great day when you hear the magic word, "REMISSION". I have a long way to go yet, but I will fight now as much as I can. I want to live, but if I do give up, I will tell you here first but first, one day at a time.

The time is now 10.30am and I have done what was an expedition to have a shower, balance in the shower and trying to climb out. Then I have to rest before I simply return to the bedroom. I am so, so wiped out now. No energy at all, not even enough to walk the short distance from the toilet and shower back to the bedroom. After 20 minutes I was able to walk to the bed. I was clean and shaven but my rash was very sore. From now on I will probably have to use an electric razor as the wet shave hurts my skin and the rash. The rash this morning is now also spotty on my chest and shoulders as well as my face and neck. So let me take note for now with me as it stands and what I have put up with from treatment ... TIRED, NO ENERGY, RASH IN FACE, CHEST, NECK, SHOULDERS, VOMITING, SWEATY, VERY COLD IN BODY, METALLIC TASTE WITH DAMAGED TASTE BUDS, HAIR AND NAIL DAMAGE, SORE TOES CAUSED BY INGROWING TOE NAILS, STOMACH PAINS, CRYING AND FEELINGS OF DEPRESSION... It is now just before 12 noon and after my absolutely awful mission to get dressed into comfortable clothes. I then returned to the toilet and promptly vomited again. I was forced to kneel over the toilet bowl and into the usual position of puking up, I had no choice but to allow the little contents of my stomach to leave my body and after the initial splash of vomit, the rest followed. I was pumping sweat but that did not stop or interrupt my violent vomiting session that went on for 15 to 20 minutes. When I finished the sweat was literally dripping off my face. I remained kneeling there while nothing happened. I had no choice as I was wiped out. After a further 10 minutes resting, I managed to stand upright and went to the bathroom nearby and washed my face etc. After that expedition, I managed to do the next expedition and negotiate the stairs downstairs. I just got to the sofa and remained there and then took all my heart and skin medication. For my rash I am now on Doxycycline and Aveeno cream. I was on Aveeno cream but then Guys followed up with an email to my doctors surgery for Doxycycline. Time will tell if it works or not. Anyhow I remained on the sofa for the afternoon. Some of my neighbours dropped me in some milk. As regards food, no food. I also have a Gastric Band at the moment which is tightened full so solid food is a no no, anyhow it tastes metallic and I am taking Fortisip drinks for nourishment. My Fortisip drinks are each with 300 calories and my favourite flavours are Apricot, Strawberry and Banana. Ginger nut biscuits are also good at getting rid of the metallic taste. I haven't tried them yet, too bloody busy vomiting. Anyhow I will try to write tomorrow as it's near 7pm and I have that epic stairs journey to make yet and we all now how long that could take and what it entails before I end up in bloody bed. Good Night all. Tomorrow is another day and it will be sometime early morning depending on how much sleep I get tonight... so, GOOD NIGHT. XXX.

——— # # # ———

HI ALL. It is THURSDAY MARCH 13TH 2014. Good morning all. I'm still in bed recovering from an earlier vomiting expedition to the toilet. When I got there I then had to play the toilet bowl waiting game. My toilet bowl has become such a good friend of mine, I can turn up at it at any time day or night unannounced and all it does is lie there while I kneel or lie in front of it. I don't kneel and pray, no, I'm different, I kneel and puke. It's an unusual combination kneeling and puking but it works for me. My normal procedure every or most mornings is as follows. This morning for example with this stage of my cancer and its associated Chemo treatment. I have woken sometimes at 1am, sometimes 2am, but so far mainly the same as any early morning human being unless you're a movie star and mornings are all great and lovey dovey, bollox. I am a normal person, so far. I take in the temperature around me and put one foot out of the bed on the ground. I generally have severe cramp in my right leg but sometimes the left one. Crippling it certainly is. I step out and put weight on that right leg or as the case may be both legs after a while it eases but only a little. I stand up and My God, the pain is awful all over and my entire body feels rough and I feel sick, so bloody sick. I took anti-sickness last night and now again but it rarely works fully or properly so some vomiting is likely to happen. The cramp soon goes as I shuffle to the toilet bowl, so far so good. I kneel like so many of those facing their doom in the Tower of London at executioners block. I wait but never disappoint. Yes you guessed correctly, projectile vomiting begins, followed by sweats. I'm dizzy, lonely, pained and no matter how long it takes, the only fluid left in me is probably in my bladder and the sweat that is now dripping from me. I sweat so much, it reminds me every time that the last time I sweated so much like this was on May 13th 2007 when I had a massive heart attack. That was hell, but once. This is hell but repeated every bloody day mainly in mornings, but sometimes a couple of times a day. Eventually I get enough courage to realise that for now the vomiting is at a halt. After gaining enough strength I then go slowly to the bathroom next door and freshen up with tooth brushing, maybe shave but definitely a shower or wash of some kind. As the Chemotherapy takes hold of my body, I feel like shit but I know that it is killing off the cells in my body, good cells and bad cells. Some cells are damaged by the chemo beyond repair and like the cancer, the bad cells are being killed off. Good cells will eventually come back. My cancer is very aggressive and sneaky. Some cancer cells will hide in the area of damaged but recoverable cells and this is where they hide and wait to come back. This is where a person in remission will suddenly find themselves with cancer again. Anyhow, I cannot tell you how important it is to have a wash regularly. It is that feeling of knowing you have cancer but you feel so, so clean again and ready to take on the day. It doesn't matter that a patient goes back to bed again after having a wash, the main thing is that it is so nice to wash the sweat and vomit off me .... Next today I weighed myself and I am just about 84 kilos. I have lost 5 kilos, about 10 lbs in the past 3 weeks. That's about 3.5 lbs per week. I have to try and take more Fortisip drinks. I eventually get to my bedroom and after the shower put on clean underwear, clean vest and basically anything else to keep warm in, including a black dressing gown. I then decided to do the trip downstairs to my sitting room. It was just as I got to the second step that I felt sick. I immediately returned to the toilet bowl and promptly vomited some more. All the running about had churned up my insides so it was easy to make me sick. I remained there hanging over the toilet bowl and then the bloody mobile phone rings. I didn't answer it as I have yet to master the art of talking and vomiting at the same time. I dare say that this particular talent has been mastered by someone somewhere. Anyhow moving on boys and girls. I finished my toilet duties and again washed my face, negotiated the stairs down in stages of descent. Twenty-five minutes later I am downstairs. The clock is now 1.20pm. I intend to take it easy for the rest of today. Today, I am going to Google conservatories. I would like a conservatory at the back of the house. It's only an idea now, but it's a good one and I need to keep my brain stimulated and plan for the future. That's another piece of advice from me, always keep your mind as positive as possible with plans for the future. Cheerio all, I will write later in the evening if I can around bedtime, so see you all then ... HELLO AGAIN, It's been a day of mixed feelings and reactions. In late afternoon my neck rash got itchy a little bit extra and very red. I am taking all the correct medication and creams and still it's as bad as ever, very itchy dry and flaky skin. Right now it's time to take on board some fluids etc in their sealed containers and bag them. After taking 10 minutes to catch my breath, it's time to climb those stairs in stages to brush my teeth. After 25 minutes, I am in my bed and Radio switched on to Classic FM. It was all hell but it had to be done. My daily routine now is controlled by the clock. The correct timings ensures that I am not getting sick for the wrong reasons. I take my medicines and intend to be asleep soon. Goodnight then all, until tomorrow.

——— # # # ———

GOOD MORNING ALL. It's Friday March 14th 2014. I must have drifted off to sleep about 9pm, as it is now 1.30am and I have the most awful pain in my head and right leg. Something new, ringing noises in my ears and these have never happened before. When I say ringing, it's a combination of ringing noises and like water droplets gurgling in my ears, both ears. It happens now and again but I have no idea when it starts and when it finishes. I have been warned about it and it could go on for days on end and may even go on in my sleep. It is sometimes unbearable as it seems like someone creating these noises inside my head. At the moment, no noises so am making the most of it and going to get some sleep .... Oh My God ... It is 6am and I am awake, very much awake. I have woken to a strange feeling of being wet on my face and chin. It is a warm wetness and going from being sleepy to wide awake in a matter of seconds because of this feeling of wetness on face and chin is strange and scary. First I thought is it a dream, but I soon realised that it was not. If this was a movie scene the camera would pan back and take in the scene. I now also feel wet on my pillow and on the bed clothes. Yes ... it is blood, lots and lots of it. I look around me and the pillow and part of the sheet is glistening wet and red from blood, I wiped my face and blood is on my hands. I am lying in my own blood and I for now have no idea where it's coming from. I got out of bed and after putting on my bedside light, I anxiously peeped at the mirror while having an idea where this blood is coming from. The mirror confirmed that blood was coming from my nose and was sourced from my left nostril. I looked back at the mess of red on my bed and realised my treatment reaction had taken a new direction, this was my first nose bleed and it all happened while I was asleep, for how long I do not know but was for a long time going by the blood loss and the mess on my bed. This new direction of treatment reaction shocked me. I was told about it but really was never prepared for it when it happened. Nose bleeds will be part of the course for my 3 drug Chemo combination reactions. Because my Chemo is more than normal, my reactions will be varied and nasty, but I did not expect them as nasty and as such so soon as this. Waking up covered in blood and lying in a bed of blood is scary. I soon realised that as soon as I recover mentally and physically today, I will shower etc and after all is done get downstairs and dump the sheet and pillowcases. No point in washing these. I will first have to change my bed into new sheet and pillow cases. For all I know it may happen again tonight but I have replacements ready on hand. Planning ahead saves a lot of embarrassment and a lot of extra shit that I don't need right now.

With all that is going on and my daily, sometimes hourly struggle with exhaustion and weariness after the slightest exertion, I now have to allow so much time for washing, laundry, climbing and descending stairs, getting about, taking medication and just putting up with everything, I sometimes have not enough time in the day to do some things after my vomiting sessions. Vomiting takes up so much time as does random bleeding, all the cleaning up afterwards, was not on my planning schedule when I was diagnosed. Nobody is prepared one way or another for what happens. I have no control over these reactions. Like crying, no control over it. I now cry several times a day. I hate crying as sometimes it's only a release of tears lasting a minute or so. A huge build up and then all hell is let lose. I have no bother in telling you that it doesn't concern me when I cry. I cry with people and when I'm alone. My crying has led me to realise that it does not show a weakness in a person. My crying has led me to be sitting alone and thinking. I don't just do this at home. The day that I was diagnosed, I cried in front of the Consultants entire team. That cry was a demented uncontrolled cry. It was a cry that separated me from everyone around me. It was also a cry that made people around me aware. As regards that diagnosis on that fateful day, the team member that told me instantly knew that from my crying she had in a couple of words destroyed my world and that of my family. To her I was just another patient, a person with an NHS number and a Hospital number. I was not the first person's life that she had changed and I was not going to be the last. After our exchange of words, I left and continued crying out into the waiting room. As I handed my appointment letter to the front desk staff, many people saw me crying. The girl that I handed the letter to then automatically knew from the list of next appointments that my crying was not for positive reasons. Her tone of voice then also automatically changed to that of a person with a voice tone suited to my reason for crying. I hope I am making sense of what I am trying to convey to you. As I said, still in

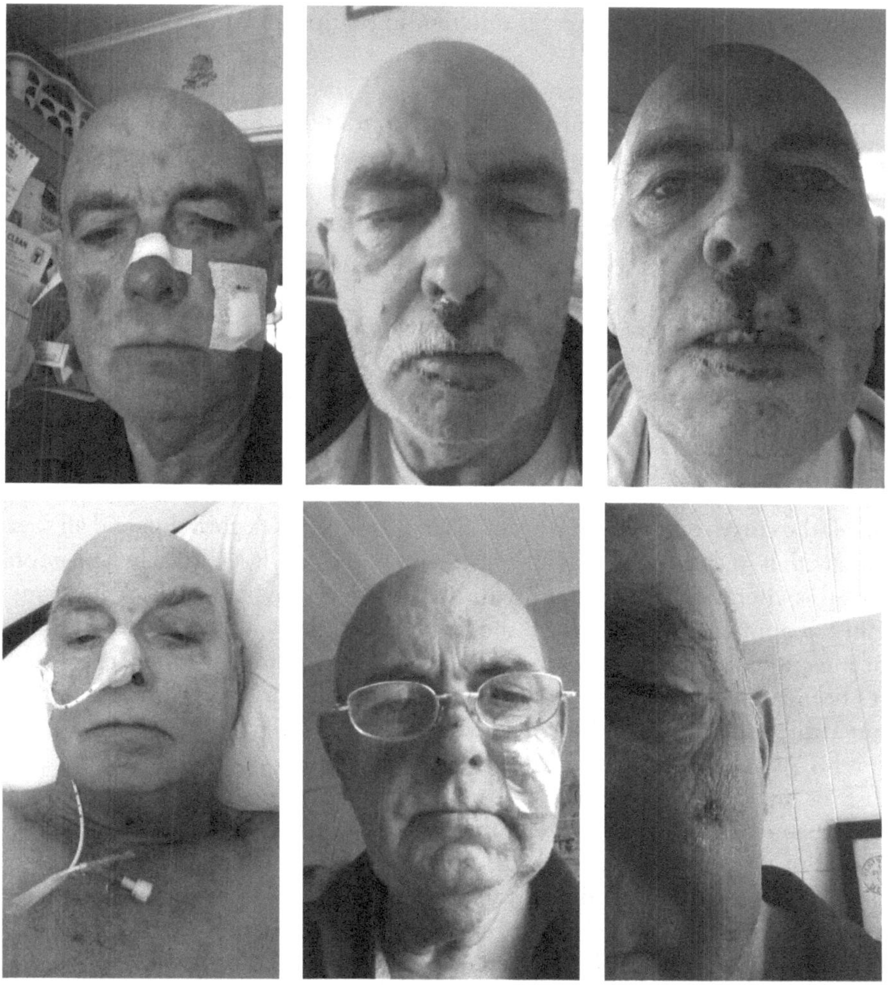

The various reactions from the Chemo.

the same waiting room were many, many people who saw me crying. They only saw me crying but have no idea whatsoever why I am crying. To them it may be either bad news (which it was) or good news like remission or the all clear. However, as we all know cancer automatically goes with bad news. The good news rarely happens but thankfully is now happening more and more. Because I look reasonably healthy at the moment and my face is new in the waiting room then most people here in the same room will assume that my crying is because of bad news. Also the family members with me are either crying or close to crying automatically allows people to decide for themselves that I am the patient in this situation. So there you go, crying can mean so little and so much. Crying out in the street is different in that people think you're crackers and treat you as so.

So now that I have taken apart the art of crying and sobbing, tears and screaming, its meanings and reasons, the right and wrong places to cry in, I promise you that I will not even attempt to explain the art of vomiting in as much detail. However, as it means you are unwell and as most people look at you vomiting, they decide for themselves that you have probably had some form of food poisoning. One thing that does make me laugh is that when you are puking your guts onto a floor or into a toilet bowl, if there are other people around me at the time, someone will always ask you "ARE YOU ALRIGHT" when it is very clear that you are not alright and you cannot speak or tell them so. That my friends is my lot on vomiting, but I can promise you one thing that when all this treatment is over, I will be an expert in the art of vomiting and crying, trust me. I am now going to get myself sorted and eventually teeth brushed, body showered, shaving done being careful with the rash and cream on all the current rash covered areas. Then it's the stairs negotiation and all that goes with it in getting downstairs for the rest of the day. It's a little after 12 noon and this afternoon or evening my district nurse is due here to disconnect my Chemo pump of 5FU and flush the line out while also checking for any signs of infections anywhere in my body. When the nurse has gone and up to now it's been a female nurse, I will write again. I have no idea when the visit is due but I will write to you all here again later …

HI AGAIN! The time is just after 11pm and that is the time this bloody district nurse turns up to disconnect my 5FU pump etc, check for infections and flush it all out. It is not the fault of the actual nurse, but it is that of those allocating the visits. I am tired and Guys Hospital Oncology have told them that to help me in my tiredness issue, I should get a late evening visit so that I can get to bed. Also there is a danger that if there is Chemotherapy liquid still in the pump, it is still going into me past the cut off point. I was promised a call for 16.00 hours to 16.30 hours, to me and you 4pm to 4.30 pm. I asked not to be late because the treatment has destroyed me now and will continue to make me even worse. Over the week the level has built up in me and over time so much chemo has now gone into my body, a body now wrapped in pain and destruction which even though is important in its job to attack my cancer, it is also destroying me. There is now a huge scary amount of chemicals going around my blood vessels and capillaries in every part of my body. Do I feel like it's doing good? No I don't. I feel like crap so who knows. As for the District nurses, they are so short staffed now, that there lies the reason why they get to me late at night. I am now ready for my bed. My PICC Line is okay so the next nurse visit is due in three weeks time for a disconnection. On my next trip to Guys Oncology they will check for infections while I am in the hospital having my one single chemo trip on Monday next coming up. I will in 3 weeks time again request an early visit and Oncology will do the same because by then I will be feeling even far, far worse. After she had made her report and left, now it's my time to do that stairs trip to my bed. Downstairs, one thing that has annoyed me is that my lovely dining room area has now been altered a little to hold a little storage area for all my drug and dressings etc associated with my cancer and chemotherapy treatment stuff. I have no choice as I need to be able to get hold of my meds easily and even maybe at very short notice. It's a shame but needs must! A box for dressings, a box for old medications, As more medications are added, then it's a new box. I have no idea if that is the case with other cancer sufferers but it is for me. I will write again in 45 minutes after I do the stairs up and get the toilet visit out of the way. It is now 11.55pm, near midnight. All is done, felt a little sick but didn't encourage things so I left the toilet as soon as I could. The stairs is my biggest obstacle and that has not changed. I cannot describe to you the agony I now go through every time I use those stairs to go up or down, but climbing is the most difficult painful event in my daily routines. I have also now decided to get something next week that I never thought I would need, yes, I need a walking stick to get around. It is getting very difficult now to get about so I need something to support my walking. I also do not know how long I will need it for but I need one, hopefully not long term. I have taken on board bottles of fluid for the night. Earlier I took on all my medications. Next Monday coming it's Guys Oncology Cancer Day Unit for 2.30pm and Cetuximab infusion over 3 hours and also a blood test. Goodnight all and as I now transfer all my diary contents onto paper, it is now past midnight and is therefore Saturday morning March 15th 2014...

——— # # # ———

GOOD AFTERNOON ALL. YES afternoon, Since I got up at 10.30am it's been non stop. I got a bad cramp in my right leg and had to walk it off or should I say hobble it off or shuffle it off. I shuffled off to the toilet back and forth and of course in the return trek to the toilet bowl I had to make it a pit stop in that I hugged the toilet bowl like I was in love with it. I soon learned that this love affair was going to be long term for many months yet to come. Today it was not the greatest place in the world to be in but, for now that was it. I puked into it for 20 minutes, then I sat on the edge of the bed for a further 30 minutes, sweating, thinking and for some unknown reason without warning, crying. As I cry without warning, I dread the day when this crying may lead to a complete mental breakdown because of the shit I'm in. It can only be a short time away. This morning also I then do my bit of planning for the day which involves negotiating that stairs. The time it takes me now is down in stages in 20 minutes and up in stages 40 to 45 minutes. That's an hour of my day just on the stairs alone. After teeth brushing, showering etc, the usual, I got downstairs about

12.10 in the afternoon. It's afternoon and the day is gone. The rest of the day was thinking and chilling out. Thinking is dangerous. Bad things enter the mind when I think. Am done now, nothing more today apart from early on later climbing those stairs and eventually some fortisip, liquids and bed. I will write again tomorrow, God willing. xx.

——— # # # ———

Hi all, It is SUNDAY MARCH 16TH 2014 and I will just quickly recap what happened today. As my condition gets worse now, my only writing now may be to recap what has happened to me in the day. Thank you for understanding but it is really wasting my body and mind now and I may not even write for some days at a time. At 7am violent vomiting happened and I never made the bowl. My vomit is on bed clothes and on the floor. I will clean it up later. I cried loud about my situation and I feel so, so alone today. I cried for nearly one hour. I finished crying and cleaned myself fully and went downstairs. While downstairs my daily lonely depressing existence was crying, thinking, sleeping, more crying, sweating and taking medications. Sorry, will write again tomorrow. Later will be getting upstairs etc and by now you know the routine better than I do. Tomorrow it's Guys for my Cetuximab infusion at 2.30 pm with blood test beforehand. It is also St Patrick's Day tomorrow. Goodnight all.

——— # # # ———

Hi everyone. It is Monday March 17th. Happy St Patrick's Day to all and it's the start of another week. I will write as it goes along for today, okay, I need to be in Guys later for my all inclusive wristband which entitles me to one infusion of Cetuximab. For things to go smoothly, I need to get there by 1.30pm to have that blood test and get results back early enough without delaying treatment. A low blood count stops treatment until it improves. Anyhow for now it's the morning routine of anti-sickness medication which should lessen the vomiting a little bit. I will write in a bit after showering, shaving and the expected vomiting, then of course there is the exhaustion of it all. I need to do all that I do upstairs because once I do that stairs trip downstairs, that's it until tonight when I go back up the stairs to bed, all 14 steps of that stairs ... Hello again, it's 11.30am, cab is on the way for my train to Guys Hospital near London Bridge. So many things are now starting to take so much longer to plan ahead, to do them and get them out of the way. You can see my morning routine takes hours to plan and implement before I tackle the stairs. The stairs is now the big ultimate dividing line in my day to day routine. Even though today is St Patricks Day, sorry but I will not be dressing up in green for the day, but Happy St Patricks Day to you all. Before that cab arrives, I have to take it easy and stop to think. I know thinking is dangerous but it does help me a lot. I have a big day ahead of me with this infusion treatment ahead of me so I will write this evening when I am home and it's all out of the way ...

Hi, I am home, been a long day but I am settled watching TV. I got to Guys for 1.20pm, plenty of time to do my people watching and my sickness diagnosis based only on watching people coming and going past me as I sat down in the hospital foyer near the coffee and snacks area, nothing but fun but it passes the day away. I went to the 10th floor The Cancer Day Unit and started the usual routine, handed over my appointment card and got the wristband. I asked if I was having a blood test, the answer was "no". No blood test today and you can bet if I was late, they would ask for a blood test, my luck! At 2.45pm I was called into one of the cubicles for treatment. Today was Zone C and I think it was a seat in the corner. I have to tell you that it is a very strange feeling every time I come in here and it is the same for every person here for treatment. The walk to the Zone C probably took a couple of minutes at most but every time my mind goes into slow motion, I look around me and every person here, all ages are all in effect here because a couple of bags of clear liquid chemotherapy in effect gives us all hope of life or an extra couple of months to live and maybe get some time to complete plans and only a few months extra is needed. It is very, very strange feeling even for those that are here to support the sick patients. For so, so many people will proceed through life and they will not even know that a place like this exists. They are the lucky people who go through life unscathed by serious sickness. I was one of those people and now look at me, 18 months to live all of a sudden and so depending on every one of these clear bags of liquid chemicals. Take for example, 18 weeks of Chemotherapy, 6 cycles and each cycle is 3 weeks. How many bags is that of Chemotherapy chemicals alone not counting the saline etc which averages 2 per session. Then there are the bags of Piriton of one per session. Altogether for the 18 weeks which for now is approximate is as follows 36 bags of saline fluid, 18 bags of Piriton and Chemotherapy is in total (5 per cycle) 30 bags. Thirty bags of Chemotherapy just for me alone. Then I get to my armchair and my slow motion thinking and reflection is over until the next time. I met Alex from my previous session here and my God that poor kid really looks so ill. A young man with a young wife and young kids and he is struck down in the prime of his life with his whole world ahead of him. I briefly spoke to him and he has deteriorated so much since we spoke last. This cancer really does not give a shit, young or old, rich and poor, male and female, it just destroys all that it touches. Alex is the proof of this. We only spoke for a few minutes as his session was over and his family were anxious to get him home. He was really fed up and like me, he said how he feels so much a burden on people. It's the same old story, everyone says that they are here for me if I need them, but, the true test is when it comes to the crunch, 20% of people are just pure and utter f*****g fakes. The remaining 80% of people are pretty genuine but of them there are still a few who are sometimes never fully truthful in their feelings. I find fakes all the time, every day, every bloody day and even in my distant family there are some, but it's such a shame. I have already said this before in my writing, but it hurts me every time because it happens all the time, every day I see it. Today also, I only spotted one patient wearing the headgear resembling a jockey, you know the one with the circulating cold water to prevent hair loss during Chemotherapy treatment. The various consultant team doctors were popping in and I had a visit from my one to check on my rash. My rash has not improved so I soon expect something else to be added to my medication mix. I was told that they would do nothing until after my consultant visit on Wednesday March 19th 2014, a couple of days away from now. I am looking forward to seeing Theresa my consultant, she is good and means well. I know that I will have a blood test today.

The visit to Theresa was exactly that and it went reasonably well in the circumstances. She looked at my rash and issued me a prescription for skin medication as expected. I left the meeting reasonably happy in view of what I am going through. I had the blood test before my meeting with Theresa. The week progressed and on Monday March 24th after my chemotherapy treatment and getting home, I had my will altered again to be up-to-date and look after my closest family. I have changed and altered this will so many times. I have made no changes to it but basically got it up to date. No doubt I will do it again at a later date to make double sure. Most people do not worry about making or changing wills but when you have a potential death sentence hanging over you, that is when it becomes so important to get it right. I had it arranged for 7pm but knew I would be home late so had it done after 9pm when the agent for will writing came to my home. All is now sorted. On Wednesday March 26th, I flew to Razgrad to be with Milena. By the time I came back on Sunday March 30th, I was getting used to the idea that this relationship was not progressing like I expected and it was all down to my poor health. On Monday March 31st, I had no treatment. On Friday APRIL 4th 2014, A district nurse came to flush out my PICC line etc. Because of the rash etc, no treatment again on Monday April 7th 2014. On Monday April 14th 2014, I had three chemotherapy drugs, back to normal treatments again. On Tuesday 15th, next day I was back in Guys for a blood test at 1pm which was followed by a blood transfusion. Good eh! They took blood from me which told them that I needed blood? I am now very, very sick and next day I returned to have another blood transfusion. My sickness got worse and now this is Day two without food or drink. Thursday 17th still at home and still very, very sick and very weak. A district nurse came to me on Friday 18th and disconnected the chemotherapy pump and then she flushed out the PICC line. Still no food or drink and my situation was really bad now. On Tuesday April 22nd, I was admitted to Guys Hospital today after treatment which was delayed by a day from yesterday. I was now in safe hands and I recovered a little enough to be discharged on April 24th. I was glad to be home and near normal eating etc, but somehow, I did not feel fully okay. On 28th there was no chemotherapy but on Wednesday 30th they gave me one drug of Chemotherapy and a pump going home pumping the drug into me. Somehow I feel that if they miss a session, then I worry that I am missing out. Monday MAY 5th 2014, No treatment. On Wednesday May 7th 2014 I had treatment drugs pumped into me and again next day with one drug. Earlier on the morning of today the 7th May, I was awake at 5.30am getting sick and hobbled to the toilet. I could feel the sick coming up from the pit of my stomach. I had cramp in my right foot, hence the hobbling to the toilet. I looked over my shoulder and noticed blood on my clothes and on the pillow and sheets. It must have happened while I slept. What followed next was a torrent of vomit and choking. I also noticed blood in my vomit which is never a good sign. My God, what next. The sweats began so I knew that I would be here for at least 30 minutes or so. Eventually after 25 minutes, I finished the vomiting I was sick and weak. I got cleaned and showered by 7am and removed the bloodied, vomit covered sheets, pillow cases and then remade my bed. I made my slow way downstairs and put the dirty sheets etc in the washing machine. Ten minutes it took to go down and put water and Fortisip into my emergency bag. The cab came and got me to the station in Orpington.

At London Bridge it was peak time. There was so many people about. I took a minute or so to stand still and people watch, busy, some looking lost, confused, drunk even this early, lonely, in love, rushing about late for whatever, running from trains, running to catch trains, suitcases going on journeys somewhere, couples holding hands, linking fingers and maybe it seems like 90% of them on mobile phones in their own world bumping into people and not an apology in sight. In the midst of all this confusion and life chaos was little me and my life is on hold. Maybe, there are more like me this morning but I am here because I want my health. I am literally fighting to stay alive, fighting to keep my balance in this fast mad world and hoping to get better so that one day I can return to take my rightful place in it. My hope to achieve this is just around the corner from here in Guy's Hospital on the 10th floor in the shape of three clear bags of Chemotherapy. These cocktail mixes are in a fridge somewhere with my name on it. I only want to live, nothing more. Surely this is not a huge demand. I eventually got to the 10th floor and soon bumped into other people on the same journey. This after all, is the 10th floor and only people with Cancer or connected to cancer in one way or another. I had the usual blood test after which followed the treatment over several hours. Gaz came to see me during his lunch break. I left shortly after 4pm with my appointment card and my wristband still attached as a reminder that I was one of the cancer filled cursed members of the human race. I was also facing that dreaded pump of 5FU attached. I think also that this is going to be the final time that it will be connected to me. I remember the day that it was first connected up to me. So much has happened since that day. I have just seen the appointment card and yes, I am back here tomorrow for one Chemotherapy drug and it will be tomorrow that the pump will be connected up to me for the final time at 11.30am. It will wreck my body but it is required to keep my treatment all up to date. Tomorrow, I will leave here happy. I got the train and then the R4 bus to near my door.

As soon I was indoors, I felt tired but after a fifteen minute rest, I quickly emptied the washing machine from the morning episode of being sick etc and hung them across the radiators. I pray that there will be no more sickness tonight. My trek upstairs took 30 gruelling minutes with breaks on the way. I took my medication and hoped for a decent night of sleep uninterrupted by any vomiting or bleeding. It is Thursday May 8th 2014 and I am all prepared for today's extra treatment at 11.30am. I do not expect any blood test today and I got there on time for my one dose of Cetuximab treatment and I was out of there by 4pm with my Pump attached. In 4 days time it will be disconnected for the last time. I got home indoors by 6pm, took on board my fluids and medication and was in bed by 8pm and obviously hoping for a sick free night and good sleep. Good morning, it is the 9th and yes, you probably guessed. I have been up since 4am with violent, weakening vomiting. It has wrenched the stomach out of me. I am sitting out looking at the weather, the road, life going by both motorised and pedestrianised. I am also looking out at my friend high up in the tree, yes Stelios my bag friend still there but hanging on for dear life, just like I am at the moment. I am staying in bed here today and I will try to write later or tomorrow. I must also stress that this is a particular nasty bout of vomiting. It is times like this that any cancer sufferer will have all the time in the world to think of his or her state of situation at present. It is at this vulnerable time that there is little to do but to convince yourself that now might be a time to reflect and think "is it all worth it". Please do not give in, giving in is too easy and this vomiting will cease eventually. There are far worse trials to come. Things will get worse, far worse before it gets any better. The treatment is worse sometimes than the cancer. This is what I have told myself and in many cases it is true. The danger is that if I am wrong after it all, I am going to look like a right proper ass. Right now I hate myself for being selected in the first place by cancer to be its host. I am the carrier of this cancer in me. I cannot contaminate anybody else, and it will probably destroy me mentally and physically, but I am determined that in time I will delay it killing me. Many people will die because of this beast of a disease. I will probably yet become one of those people. After all my prognosis is maximum of 18 months to live. The worst of this disease is having time on your hands and having too much time to think.

On the 12th a nurse came out to disconnect the pump and flush it out.

That was it, no more pump attached to me anymore. At least, that is the plan. The nurse after doing her flushing, then made her report and was in and out in 15 minutes. However, no sooner had she gone when I was very sick again. My body feels like it is shutting down. It is a horrible time now for me. I cannot even think straight or focus my mind on anything in particular. I cannot talk or make decisions for myself. Having no idea what time it is, I reached out for my pound shop glasses that were beside me and all I noticed was hearing some birds singing outside. I could not focus or see properly so I assumed it was in the afternoon. I was confused. I took some medications and for some reason went upstairs which took me at least 30 minutes to climb the stairs. I just fell onto the bed and must soon have fallen asleep. It was frightening as I had no idea what was going on around me. I suddenly awoke and I realised that it was near 10pm at night. I had also taken on board in my emergency bag some fortisips and water in bottles. I felt so low that I may not venture downstairs from this bedroom for a few days. My heating was up full and yet I was freezing. I was very, very low and could I be actually dying? Garreth was away with work and I spoke to him to tell him what was going on with me and my body. I thought a lot about dying and death. I do not want to die alone but at least people now know how bad I am and what this f*****g cancer, this bastard of a disease is doing to me. I cried and cried and cried. I was so healthy, I loved my work, my life and my friends. I loved my holidays and I adored my lovely Skiathos. I thought, if I die will there be life after death that I can go there and stay there. I cried out loud and actually now wanted to die. I cannot go on. Please God let me fall asleep and die in my sleep. Nobody else called me and the inevitable happened. Goodnight all and goodnight Stelios. I soon fell asleep and peace had entered my mind and body at last.

On Tuesday 13th May, I awoke after a good sleep but did not feel good at all. I think everybody knows when their body is showing problems and soon it may be time to go to A and E, but not yet. I was upstairs but had no reason to be here. I showered and got dressed. I went downstairs. I was not as bad and as depressed as last night but I was feeling very, very bad indeed. I went downstairs and soon realised that my emergency bag was back upstairs. I needed that bag in case I was going to hospital. I struggled back upstairs and had to lie down. I was wiped out. It was about 5pm. I awoke at 6.15pm and felt sick. I got to the toilet and just puked and puked and sweated my brains out. I went back to my bed but soon I collapsed on my bed. On recovery an hour or so later, I found myself on the floor. It was my own fault as I had not taken any water on board and I was dehydrated and felt close to the end. I recovered a little, got myself off the floor and at 11.30pm, I called an ambulance. I called Garreth and told him that I was very sick. I also told him that I was going to go to Hospital. I also told my sister Mary of my situation and my decision. I think it was the correct decision in the circumstances. I was admitted to The Princess Royal

University Hospital. I was lucky in a way that I was able to call the ambulance, because if I had not, then I may have died at home alone. After I was taken by ambulance my phone was soon busy with messages enquiring about my health. In my road, we are all such a close community that when an ambulance appears and is near a house that people know, my neighbours are asking about me. This is the one reason that I just love my road and my neighbours. I help them and they are always offering to help me. I do however worry about being sick and living alone. That is my greatest worry. Now however, I was safe in hospital. My house was secured and all I wanted was to get better as soon as possible. I was very, very sick again and dehydrated. I was hooked up to a bag of fluids as I was badly dehydrated. I thought "here we go again".

On Monday 19th I was told that I had no white blood cells and injections into my thigh were needed to boost my system. I would soon however have complications from someone making a mistake. I was put in a ward with a patient with Gastroenteritis even though my immune system was wiped out from Chemotherapy. I was however safer and avoiding infections at home so I was soon on my way home.

On the 20th, I was discharged but feeling much better. My own bed tonight. Hi to Stelios. My condition is near as good as it is going to be. Guys have been in contact with the people looking after me and my Chemotherapy which was cancelled last week has now been planned again to happen. I do not like missing out on treatment if possible. I am relieved and happy to hear that it is planned for tomorrow 21st in Guys at 2.30pm. It will be my last cetuximab drug treatment. Treatment is also planned again on 23rd at also 2.30pm. My self medication and self injecting is continuing as normal. Stelios is looking very battered in that tree. Not looking bright orange now, but still there keeping me company. I shout at him but he never argues back. After my stay in hospital, I feel reasonably good. After I got home, I managed to climb the stairs in 10 minutes from base camp to summit and during the night I had to go downstairs to reduce the heating. I managed it in 5 to 6 minutes. My condition is not bad, doing the stairs is a little easier for now, no sickness vomiting yet but I also realise that I have been doing nothing in hospital. My numbness and tingling in toes and fingers is still present as is all the other problems and chemotherapy reactions. I realise that the violent vomiting took up a lot of my time hanging over the toilet bowl for hours on end, I am concerned however that my right upper thigh area now is sore.

Hi, it is Wednesday May 21st 2014. I think back to the hospital as it is possibly there that I had a suspected dirty needle incident and I fear the worst. I escaped the gastroenteritis problem. My immune system was depleted so I fear the worst with this suspected dirty needle was at the same time with no immune system. I am going for chemotherapy later so I will speak some time afterwards. I may show my infected thigh to my treatment nurses later in Guys.

For now, it's time to get organised and do what I can here and get to Guys for Chemotherapy treatment at 2.30pm. I think it's best if I write to you later after I get home from treatment. Time now is 11am and will talk later.

Good evening all, I last spoke to you at about 11am. I got to Guys in my usual way. My walking stick was needed, this chemotherapy has messed up my joints a lot now. At Guys, I was taken for my infusion treatment in Zone C. During my three hours, I did show my right upper thigh to the nurses and was advised to go to my GP as soon as possible. While connected up in Guys I made an appointment for tomorrow morning very early at 9am with my GP about my right upper thigh. Job done. I slept as usual even though I was only there for a few hours. Gaz came to see me around 3pm and I was out of there around 6pm. I didn't hang around and on the way to the station looked up and had 5 minutes to get that train to Orpington. I got there as the train pulled in and Yes I did squeeze into it my rucksack and walking stick slotted in beside me. It beats me how people can read an Evening Standard in a packed train, but they do it. I suppose it's down to years of practice on the same commute every evening. I got to Orpington and then the bus R4 near to my front door. I was wiped out. I have not felt like this in a long time. I got indoors and suddenly noticed my right leg was very sore to touch. I had to take a look, my God there was a huge yellow blister like a bubble ready to burst. Am glad now that I'm seeing doctor in the morning at 9am. Anyhow, I got myself prepared for tonight. How quick can I do the stairs in tonight. I repacked my emergency bag with fresh new clothes etc. I had a mug of tea and some fortisip. I got my pack together and decided to have an early night. I felt a bit queasy but no major vomiting yet. I hobbled up the stairs in ten minutes. At least I'm maintaining my new personal best at this climb to the Summit. Yes I did stop on the way at stair 7 or 8. Upstairs I loaded up my little fridge with my water and Fortisip drinks. My medications too were with me and I had taken some earlier. However, I cannot forget my immune system is ripped apart at the moment so I am likely to pick any bad things up. I have to be so careful now still. Okay, no vomiting and I went to bed. It was about 9.20pm and therefore a reasonable time for bed. Goodnight all and Goodnight Stelios.

——— # # # ———

THURSDAY MAY 22ND 2014. I am sad this morning. Overnight I lost Stelios. He was there yesterday morning as I went to my treatment and it was dark last night so I assumed he was in the tree. Lately he was looking tattered and bruised but still hung in there. This morning when I looked up, I noticed that there is only a small piece of faded plastic, maybe six inches long, still there but the main part is gone, possibly blown away. My friend wrenched from me as my back was turned. Life goes on and I will not replace him. Amazing that when my main chemotherapy comes to an end, he decides to go. I also feel a little sick so it's time to take anti-sickness medicine to try to put a stop to any vomiting session planned for me. No other problems this morning apart from peripheral neuropathy in all fingers and all feet and toes. I am very, very tired, wiped out in fact but it's 7.15am and I have a 9am doctors appointment about my right upper thigh. I got downstairs in 5 minutes and left the house to get to my doctors. I was lucky to get this appointment. I saw Dr P and my leg is now a mess, an absolute mess. A large green and yellow boil that is ballooning and now leaking a little. He called the nurse, and took a swab to be sent away. The nurse in the practice lanced it and blood and yellow liquid flowed out of it and down my leg. My God what damage has been done to me by this dirty needle and the blunder. I feel sick weak and now badly infected by having no immune system. The nurse put "medihoney" on the wound and dressed it well. She then made a phone call and arranged for a District nurse to come out to me to dress the wound. The district nurse would come out to me next on SUNDAY MAY 25th 2014 to clean the wound and then every few days until all healed. Let me tell you now, look out for any mistakes by the medical people. My history with district nurses is not great but with a leg as bad as this, what is the worst that can happen apart from an amputation! District nurses probably mean well but some of them if they were on fire, I wouldn't piss on them to put the fire out. They are there to protect you and me, look what they done to me, okay it was a mistake but it shouldn't have happened. Hospitals and nurses are brilliant and when we go to hospital we depend on them to look after us. I believe if they had simply changed their clean practices, this may not have happened to me. I left the doctors and as it was only around 10am I had the rest of the day to take it easy and slowly get some housework done. My housework is well overdue and more chemotherapy tomorrow means today is the only day. Cheerio all and I will write tomorrow after my treatment so until tomorrow evening then. Cheerio.

——— # # # ———

FRIDAY MAY 23rd 2014. Hi all, just a quick word to let you know that in my local hospital the PRUH today I had a blood test. My extra treatment of chemotherapy for today in Guys was cancelled last night. I never have treatment on a Friday anyway so I do not know, maybe a typo error. This morning beforehand I had a vomiting session and a slight nose bleed but apart from the metallic taste in my mouth and the numbness and tingling in toes, feet and fingers, most things are as they were up to now. I will write again as soon as I can. District nurses are doing the monitoring of my wound in my right thigh. District nurse due here on Sunday 25th to clean the thigh wound. I will write then, cheerio all. I wonder where Stelios is now?

——— # # # ———

SUNDAY 25th MAY 2014. Hi all just to say, my district nurse arrived tonight at 8pm and dressed my leg wound. It is still very, very raw and oozing horrible stuff. She put strips of Medihoney on it to speed up its getting-better progress and no doubt a return trip. She done her report and left. I myself feel very weak, tired and also feeling very sick. Good night one and all out there.

——— # # # ———

THURSDAY 29th MAY 2014. Generally I feel crap, tired and a little depressed and lonely. When is this hell gonna end. District nurse came out this evening about 7pm, changed dressing on leg wound and told me that finally it's working and the wound is getting better. My stairs climbing has not changed, still 10 minutes going up and 5 going down. Cheerio all.

——— # # # ———

FRIDAY 30TH MAY 2014. Just a quick hello, had a phone call to say that the district nurse would be out tomorrow to change leg dressing and flush the PICC line as it's needed to keep the area clean and it's not in use at the moment while My system is having another break from Cetuxima. Cheerio all.

——— # # # ———

SATURDAY MAY 31st 2014. District nurse came out tonight at 8pm and changed dressing on my leg wound. She also flushed out my PICC Line. as this has to be done either in the home or in hospital at least once weekly. She done her work and report and left. She is returning tomorrow night again to change the leg dressing. As for my condition, this break from Cetuximab is nice. I am still having nausea but no vomiting. Loneliness is awful with some days not seeing anybody or even hearing from them. I have the feet and finger problems. It will be short lived as treatment is planned for June 28th at 2.30pm. Good day to you all.

——— # # # ———

SUNDAY JUNE 1st 2014. Nothing changed from yesterday. Just shows really what harm the treatment is doing to me. No treatment and the result is a pretty hassle free time. Anyhow, the district nurse again came out at 7pm tonight and changed the thigh wound dressing. She done her report and left after 45 minutes or so. There are no great changes to my condition. I think it's amazing how quick the leg wound is now healing. It is all down to this MEDIHONEY. Therefore I can only say that any bad cuts or infections from now on will get the Medihoney treatment and it is so quick. She left as I said after 45 minutes once her report was done and I believe that the district nurses will have one more visit on June 4th to change the dressing. She contacted my GP and made an advanced appointment for me to attend on Monday June 9th at 11.15am. I will write on Monday evening June 2nd 2014 tomorrow as I have a very important appointment at 11am. That big appointment is in St Thomas' for a PET Scan which is a deep tissue scan that seeks out the exact status of my cancer. I will write in afternoon or evening after it to explain it all. Therefore in the meantime just to tell you on my latest state of health. I still have problems with peripheral neuropathy which is tingling and numbness in toes, soles of feet and fingertips. Sometimes I have incidents of vomiting whereas in the past it was on a daily basis guaranteed, now it is mainly every second day or so but when it does happen, it is still without warning. I still need my walking stick as chemo has messed up my knee joints. I am very, very tired and this has not got better. I don't sleep much as I am always thinking why me, why did I get this f*****g disease, I still hate healthy people purely just because why me. I never done harm to anybody in my life and I am now condemned to die a horrible death and I don't know when that will happen. I am very slow still on the stairs up and down, I still have the metallic taste in my mouth and I can only take Fortisip drinks to get calories into me. The nose bleeds have eased off but as I list all of these things happening to me, I realise that they will return. The problem is that will they be as bad or worse so the main thing now is to enjoy my good days knowing that they may be short lived. Okay, I have a new annoying condition in my feet. I have very sore toenails. As you know that Chemotherapy does crazy things to hair and nails. I am seeing my GP in a few days time again and I will ask him. My biggest worry is that now more crazy things are happening and this could be ingrowing toenails etc. Lets see eh!

——— # # # ———

MONDAY JUNE 2ND 2014. Hi all, big day today for me. At 11am I have an appointment for a pet Scan. It's a deep tissue scan of the whole body and checks the exact state of my cancer. It will tell if the chemotherapy is doing its work or not. I took the train as usual but got off at Waterloo East and walked up to St Thomas' and got the lift to the PET CENTRE. This scan involves being taken in and a cannula put in my arm and after taking my details and a list of medications, I am then taken to what is called the "HOT ROOM". In this hot room, I am in a cubicle and the "Radiation sugar" is injected into me via the cannula. The cannula is then removed and I sleep or rest for the next hour and a half while this radiation is going around my body into every nook and cranny. After the 1.5 hours I am then taken in a fashion failure type of gown to the scanning room for two scans. If the fashion police caught me in this gown, I would be taken away and never seen again. First scan lasts 15 minutes of my head and neck area of my body, then I am scanned for 30 or so minutes of the rest of the body. I must tell you that fasting is recommended for 6 to 8 hours prior to the scan. I always fast from the night before to make sure. Afterwards I get dressed and wait in the waiting room having tea or coffee. One of the staff then comes out and says the images were good and I am free to go. It was a tiring day and was glad to get home. I will know on June 11th when I see Theresa next. Cheerio all.

——— # # # ———

WEDNESDAY 4th JUNE 2014. District nurse came out for the last time this evening and dressed my leg wound. As you know she has already made my appointment to see my GP and practice nurse on Monday June 9th 2014. She left after her report and is very happy with my leg wound ... That is it, cheerio all until the 9th.

——— # # # ———

MONDAY JUNE 9th 2014. Good afternoon all. been to my GP and practice nurse earlier and apart from my doctor requesting a blood test which I will have later, he looked at my leg wound with the nurse and was very pleased with its progress. The GP also looked at my toes and has referred me to a chiropodist as he believes that the chemotherapy has caused me to have ingrowing toe nails. He said that just by looking at them, at least two would possibly need surgery to be removed and a couple of more toenails at least need partial removal. The nurse in the practice dressed my thigh wound and wants to see me back here on Wednesday 11th at 9am to change dressings etc. I had my blood test in Orpington Hospital and returned home to rest. As soon as I got home I not only had a nose bleed but also had a vomiting session. Just to remind me that nothing changes and I am not out of the woods yet and yet something new to add to my ongoing problems is my legs are now very swollen which I think is fluid retention. This is the second new problem in past couple of days. I am resting for the rest of today, but on checking my calendar I will have to have a rush morning on 11th as that is the day that Theresa wants to discuss my scan results Until then, cheerio all.

——— # # # ———

WEDNESDAY. JUNE 11th 2014. Good morning, it is 7.30am and this morning I am just after having a vomiting incident but only a slight one. I suppose it was more coughing up water than vomiting. One of my toes is bleeding under the nail in my right foot. I am extremely tired, no energy, slow to get around, all things taste metal or paper, my eyes are puffy and red again so that's for the nurse this morning. I went to see my doctor after 8.45am. I showed him my eyes and again the swollen feet. My blood test came back still showing low white cell count which means the injections continue to boost my white cells and therefore my immune system. My eyes need eye drops and he gave me fluid retention tablets for the fluid retention. The nurse dressed the wound and simply asked me to come back tomorrow at 9.15am. I left and went home to rest. It had been a busy morning and I wanted to sit down and rest. I got home and took it easy. I checked my emergency bag just in case I need it in future and done some small clothes washing. I was able to use the stairs okay for now and at 1pm drove straight to Orpington Station to get to Guys for 2.40pm. I hadn't been here for a while but nothing changes. People are still sitting around people watching. I joined them as I had time to spare. At 2.30pm I went into Oncology outpatients and gave in my appointment letter. I was called for height and weight. Gaz was to meet me there and at 2.40, in he came. Then I saw the sign that Theresa's clinic was running 1 hour late. I was glad that Gaz was there and I had a good feeling about this meeting. At 3.30pm Gaz was the first to hear my name being called and then it appeared on the screen. We went into a room at the top of the corridor and there was Theresa. I sat down and she simply said, "Well, we have good news". I knew it was good. She explained that I was in Partial Remission and had a good response to the treatment. She then said that to continue the work I should take on maintenance cetuximab on a regular weekly basis to have any effect on the cancer. I didn't care, I was so relieved and so was Gaz. If this cetuximb is actually the reason for my great response to the cancer, then why not. I will have Cetuximab for breakfast, dinner and tea. I hugged everyone around me, Gaz and I hugged Theresa. What a consultant to be having such a result in keeping me on this planet. We calmed down and left the room. We left the hospital in an upbeat mood. We were both really happy now. I think Gaz went to his place and I went home to pack. Tomorrow morning was Thursday 12th and I had a 9.15 am appointment with the nurse in my doctors surgery to check my thigh wound which actually is healing up very well. I left the doctor surgery and returned home to pack a bag. Tomorrow is Friday 13th and I was making my way to Luton tonight to check into a hotel before flying out early tomorrow morning to Milena in Bulgaria. The next couple of days was going to be my time and while there it was time to reflect on my life and my cancer taking over. I travel the night before to prevent any panic or stress on Friday morning and get on a flight in a calm state of mind. The next few days were mine so I will write again after my return. This time I am spending longer than normal in Razgrad with Milena. I return into Luton from Varna on Friday June 20th.

——— # # # ———

SATURDAY JUNE 21ST 2014. Good morning all. I am home and actually feeling okay. At this stage I have no idea when I will be back in Bulgaria. I also am now beginning to fully realise that Milena and I will not last the long term. I have too much to do here in U K with my family and friends. More about that another time. Now it's time to enjoy my weekend as on Monday 23rd I am back up in Guys to have at 2.30pm a 3 hour session of maintenance cetuximab only. This is solely to keep the cancer under control for now. Cheerio all for now, we will talk again on Monday morning 23rd. Have a nice weekend everyone.

——— # # # ———

GOOD MORNING ALL. IT IS MONDAY JUNE 23rd AND IT'S TREATMENT DAY FOR ME AGAIN. I have to be in Guys for 2.30pm. It's a milestone day as it is the first day of this maintenance chemotherapy regime set out for me. I have no idea what will be the outcome but Theresa my consultant is hopeful as so far I have had a good response to treatment. My trip to Guys is the same as before, cab to Orpington Station and train to London Bridge and that struggle of a walk to the Oncology cancer treatment centre on that 10th floor. I won't bore you with the details as it's always the same now. My infusion today was in Zone C and was over in 3 hours or so. Afterwards, when all was completed, I collected my treatment appointment card and left to get to the station and home. I have no idea what lies ahead as regards reaction to treatment as I am back here again next week for more maintenance cetuximab on 30th at 1pm. From now on I have decided to write my blog differently, purely and simply because very little is actually happening now. This evening after returning home, I was vomiting a little because of treatment. However my legs are sore and I am having problems walking. It's time to see my GP as I think I have ingrowing toenails caused by my Chemotherapy treatment. That's it for today and will write next when I have that doctors appointment.

——— # # # ———

GOOD MORNING All, It is WEDNESDAY JUNE 25th 2014. I had a doctor appointment this morning at 11.20am with Dr. P. I am not sick but I do now have a problem with ingrowing toenails which is going to be very, very painful. I cannot ignore it as it's only going to get worse as time goes by. Chemotherapy does awful strange things to various parts of the body. This is just another thing that I am adding to the list of weird and wonderful things happening to my body right now. As you know it creates hair loss and weight loss, sometimes weight gain. It also speeds up the nail growth in the body. Right now it is playing hell with toe nails and speeding up their growth. My toe nails are ingrowing and need to be operated on and possibly removed. A very painful time lies ahead for me. My GP, Dr P, has seen me and is considering seeing to referring me to a chiropodist in Orpington Hospital to treat and do what is necessary as regards these toenails. On Friday at 3.45pm I had an appointment with my dietician at St. Christophers Hospice. Nothing out of the ordinary to report with the dietician but they are monitoring my condition. Tomorrow morning is going to be the beginning of a mad weekend. Julie is here from Bristol for the weekend but returning on Sunday. Tomorrow morning my brother Liam is arriving from Heathrow by car. Gaz, my pride and joy of a son, is also arriving to help me deal with everyone. I am not sick apart from feeling sick and having my toenail problems.

——— # # # ———

MONDAY MORNING. JUNE 30th 2014. Good morning all. Today peace and quite has returned. Everyone has gone home but was lovely seeing them. I have a chemo appointment this afternoon at 3pm for maintenance cetuximab. I also have an infection in my PICC line so that may be coming out today. My toes infections are bad and now I have problems walking properly. The day went well and yes my PICC line was removed due to an infection in it. From now on all treatment will be via a cannula. No problem to me at all.

——— # # # ———

MONDAY MORNING, JULY 1st 2014. I had a 12 noon appointment with my GP who took toe swabs of the problems in my toes. On Wed July 2nd my GP gave me antibiotics to treat my toe infections even though I know the problem is ingrowing toenails. On Thursday morning I went to my old place of work at New Cross Bus Garage at 1 am, to catch up with my old work mates. Had a nice morning there. Good to catch up with those that were there. July 7th at 1.30pm I had another cetuximab appointment and on Tuesday July 8th 2014 at 5.10 pm I had an appointment with my GP. On Thursday July 10th I had an appointment with the company doctor basically to get an update on my cancer and its treatment before he reports back to head office of my employers. If anyone out there wants help in this matter do not hesitate to contact me.

——— # # # ———

MONDAY JULY 14th 2014 another cetuximab chemotherapy appointment at 1.30pm. Nothing unusual to report and for the rest of this week my only appointments were on tomorrow Tuesday 15th a GP appointment and on Wednesday 16th at 10.30am an appointment with Theresa my consultant basically to check on my progress etc. My cetuximab chemotherapy appointments were as planned on July 21st at 2. 30pm and July 28th at 1.30pm. This was followed by a 10.30am appointment to see my GP on Tuesday 29th. More cetuximab chemotherapy on Monday August 4th 2014 and as you notice now it's well into summertime but I have heating on. That is what Chemotherapy does to the human body. Tomorrow is Tuesday August 5th and I have a meeting with my manager in New Cross Bus Garage. On Wednesday at 10.30am I see my consultant in Guys and on Wednesday night I travel to Luton prior to my Thursday morning early flight to Milena in Bulgaria. I have to admit I do not know how long this long distance relationship is going to continue for. On Saturday August 9th, while in Razgrad in Bulgaria, things changed dramatically for me. All my toes were now tingling. A lot of my toenails are now bleeding in both feet. They are all tingling and I am now very worried for my general health again after having a number of weeks of no problems.

——— # # # ———

ON MONDAY AUGUST 11th 2014 things dramatically changed when I had blurred vision. Also this week is the 1st Anniversary of Milena and I meeting. All this week Milena and I are on a beach on the Black Sea coast near Varna. On Friday 15th the problems continued where I totally lost my sight. There is nothing, nothing more scary than losing eyesight completely. By late evening my sight was returning and on Sunday evening 17th August, I was glad to return home to Luton from Varna. In all a total of 8 toenails are now continually bleeding and as yet no referral to see a chiropodist about the problem which is now getting far, far worse by the day

——— # # # ———

On MONDAY AUGUST 18th my maintenance chemotherapy cetuximab resumed. All day, every day, every hour, the bleeding and tingling toes continued relentless. More cetuximab chemotherapy on Tuesday August 26th (date change) also with a blood test on the same day. Everything up to now was going so well that a few months ago I actually wanted to go back to work and tomorrow at 11am a meeting was arranged to make a decision one way or the other if I was returning to work or not. However, my bleeding toes etc has put paid to that and now management are drawing up final figures to pay me off with a medical dismissal sometime and a suitable financial final pension package etc. My bleeding toes are relentless as is a new bad problem now of Peripheral Neuropathy. This is having no feeling whatsoever in fingers and toes. After months of good life, my life is in utter turmoil again. A letter from my employers has gone to DVLA to inform them of my employers medically dismissing me. I was hoping against hope but hidden problems keep popping their heads up and who knows what is about to show its ugly head and how soon that will happen. Too good to be true but Hey Ho!

——— # # # ———

MONDAY SEPTEMBER 1ST 2014 maintenance chemotherapy Cetuximab at 2pm. Tomorrow at 9.30am I have a Pet Scan in St Thomas' Hospital, it's the usual one where radiation sugar is pumped into me over a period of a few hours. My consultant will have the result on her desk tomorrow morning but I have to wait until Wednesday 10th September 2014, basically next week. My toes continue to bleed every day and my peripheral neuropathy which is tingling and numbness is really back with a vengeance. Tomorrow, Wednesday, I am at my old place of work, New Cross Bus Garage to see my Garage management and what they are possibly going to offer me as I expect a promising completion of my employment settlement agreement soon. Do not get me wrong, I was a good employee and I expect my pension settlement to be agreeable to me when the time comes. My toes and peripheral neuropathy continue to be a very major problem right now.

——— # # # ———

MONDAY SEPTEMBER 8TH 2014, I have Chemotherapy at 1.30pm ... yes the usual maintenance cetuximab. Tomorrow I have an appointment with my GP to get referred to a chiropodist sorting out my toes and their problems. My doctor has told me to expect painful times ahead as the toe nails are ingrowing and the only solution is lots of cutting and full removal of some nails. Not an easy thing to face on top of the bloody cancer but right now it's affecting my walking and generally day-to-day getting around.

——— # # # ———

WEDNESDAY SEPTEMBER 10TH 2014, big day today and guess what happened. At 5.40pm I had an appointment with Theresa my consultant to get my pet scan results and basically, with Gaz beside me, Theresa told me that I was in remission. Cancer is on hold and stable and all because of Cetuximab. Therefore to maintain this progress the cetuximab will continue. I am so, so happy, it's a strange feeling to be told that for now I have bought extra time and life is great right now. I left the room and stepped out a strange man. Earlier I walked in facing death and now I had bought extra time to do some more things in my life. Could never have dreamed this earlier in the day, just shows, you never know what any day can bring to your life .

——— # # # ———

THURSDAY SEPTEMBER 11TH my union advised me to appeal the company decision to medically dismiss me. Basically it's my legal right as regards employment law and in the meantime my employer still pays me something while my appeal goes through. The union lodged the appeal on my behalf.

——— # # # ———

FRIDAY SEPTEMBER 12th 2014. I now have another annoying problem which is a terrible rash on my face, this is on top of my other issues of bleeding toe nails ingrowing and peripheral neuropathy.

——— # # # ———

MONDAY SEPTEMBER 15th. My gastric band was checked out today. It's no longer got restriction but while it's there it has to be checked out and my weight is now levelled out. My rash is now all over chest and face this week after spreading to my chest. Where next? The problems continue without ease, no let up at all. More chemo on 22nd and on Saturday 27th my retired pass arrived. This is before the company had listened to my appeal. Talk about jumping the gun but at least I got my retired company pass from them. More chemo on 29th and on Saturday October 4th 2014 I had my flu jab in the morning. Great isn't it, I have this f*****g cancer and they give me a jab to prevent me getting flu. xx ha ha.

——— # # # ———

SATURDAY OCTOBER 5th I travelled to Milena in Bulgaria to celebrate my 57th birthday there. My chemo on Monday is cancelled to give me a break which then allows me to do these trips abroad. As a birthday treat in Razgrad I visited the club of LUDOGORETS in Razgrad and their training ground.

——— # # # ———

SATURDAY OCTOBER 12th, I arrived home from Bulgaria. I honestly do not know how long these trips will last now. Cracks are appearing and to be honest, I am not too bothered. My life and family are here as well as my treatment.

——— # # # ———

ON WEDNESDAY OCTOBER 15th, I had an appointment with Dr. K********at 9am to check my heart, so far so good. In the afternoon in Guys at 2.20pm, I saw Theresa my consultant just to check me out. At this stage many things were suddenly about to have dramatic events in my life,

——— # # # ———

ON SUNDAY, yes Sunday OCTOBER 19th, I was called into the Princess Royal University Hospital for an ECHO TEST at 1.00pm. The next morning was Monday October 20th 2014 and strangely my mobile phone rang. I was immediately advised to stop everything and slowly, without rushing, make my way to Cardiology in the PRUH. I was told to contact family and the advice was that they had discovered clot in my heart and it had to be dispersed quickly as there was a danger of a heart attack and possible death. On arrival I was admitted and was told that a treadmill test which was planned would now obviously be cancelled to avoid any stress to my heart. I was then told that there were 2 clots in my heart. Strangely my appeal for my employers to reconsider their decision to medically dismiss me was also on today.

——— # # # ———

TUESDAY OCTOBER 21st 2014. Reluctantly I made two phone calls, one to my union official in Merton expecting me to be in attendance and I told him that I was in the PRUH after having 2 clots in my heart. If I did have any hope of coming back, my fate was now sealed. My second call was to DVLA to tell them also the same facts of what happened. Tomorrow is WEDNESDAY OCTOBER 22nd 2014 and my God I could never imagine what was lying ahead for me. Things were bad now, they were about to get far, far worse ....

——— # # # ———

Hi all, it's WEDNESDAY OCTOBER 22nd 2014. By the time this day would come to an end my life would have taken another drastic change. The day started well, just a normal morning in a hospital. I had come to terms with the fact that I had two clots in my heart and the worry that at any moment one or even both of these clots could break away and possibly kill me. Having put in my appeal at work yesterday, my sole purpose now was to get my pension deal sorted out to benefit me. I also expected today sometime that my union rep would come to me with a pension offer. I now realise that these heart clots have well and truly put my return to work idea straight into the bin, This morning also, I was told by the nurse in charge that I was to be taken to Guys for a Cardiac MRI Scan. By early evening I was back in the PRUH and awaiting Gaz coming to see me with his then girlfriend who I was to meet for the first time. John, my union rep, was on the way but Gaz and his girlfriend arrived first. It was lovely meeting her. John then arrived at 7.30 pm with my pension offer in writing. I hesitated for a while but realised that I had to accept which is what I did and told him so to get the company to draw up the appropriate necessary contracts for me to sign in acceptance. This would be it, accepting a pension etc to live on for whatever time I got left with this cancer unless my bad heart gets me first. John my union rep left. We carried on chatting but I immediately noticed that I was feeling sick and sweaty. I soon realised that this was not looking good and I asked Gaz to get a nurse and to tell her that I thought I was slowly having a heart attack. I could not believe it. Here I am and I soon realised the signs were there. A nurse came and arranged an ECG on my heart. Soon it was confirmed that I was having a heart attack and his girlfriend was meeting me for the first time and had to look at me having a heart attack right in front of her. I was made comfortable and given the necessary medication to help my situation. Gaz and his then girlfriend left and I was told that next morning I was to be taken to Kings College Hospital for possible stents to be inserted if the situation needed it. Well what a f*****g day that was. What next is in line for me to face in my ongoing cancer battle. I am however pleased with the offer that the company made to me. For the next few days I just spent my time in hospital getting rest and relaxation. I cannot believe that I have had another heart attack.

——— # # # ———

On WEDNESDAY OCTOBER 27th 2014 my Chemotherapy in Guys was cancelled. My left middle toe is bleeding badly and from a burst blister on the left side of my stomach, On Tuesday 28th there was a virus in Medical 8 so all treatments due to me did not happen. I had a blood test and been told that the clots are dispersing as planned. My union rep called me to say that the appropriate forms had been drawn up and all I had to do when they arrived was to sign and return. It would be hard to do and in effect would be signing my work life away. End of an era eh. Angiograms planned for Wednesday 29th and Thursday 30th were both cancelled as it meant transporting me by

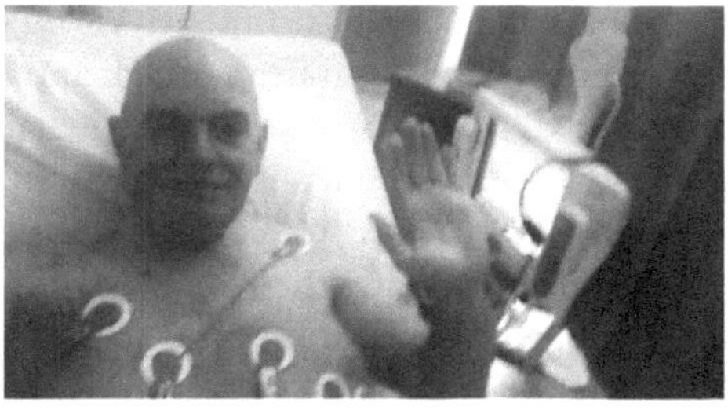

October 2014 when I had my heart attack.

ambulance that were not available for one reason or another. I am feeling totally exhausted for what has happened over past few days etc. Finally the long awaited angiogram happened in the morning of today

——— # # # ———

FRIDAY 31st October 2014. I did not have any stents inserted and later in the afternoon my day in Kings came to an end. I was returned to the PRUH and apart from being very very tired, I was told that tomorrow SATURDAY NOVEMBER 1st 2014 that I might be going home. I was discharged. from the Princess Royal University Hospital. I remain tired and again on MONDAY NOVEMBER 3rd my Chemo in Guys was cancelled. Tuesday November 4th at 9am I attended the warfarin clinic in the PRUH. On Wednesday 5th November, I went to see Theresa my consultant in Guys at 2.40pm. I was able to make the journey by train to London Bridge and then the short walk to Guys Hospital. So many times I now make this same journey to Guys for treatment and visits like this to see Theresa Guerrero-Urbano or a member of her team. So far they have really done so well to keep me alive, not necessarily healthy but still a short but safe distance from the undertaker. Sorry Mr Uden my undertaker, but no business from me as yet. On arriving at Guys, I went to the Oncology Out Patients waiting room and checked in as before. Soon Garreth my son who attends all these consultant appointments with me noticed my name on the screen for blood testing and weight checking. I returned to the waiting room after the weigh in and the blood test and with Gaz we both waited for my name to again appear on screen which this time would be to see Theresa or the team. As before, I always wanted to see Theresa herself as she always gave me good news. Today, according to the screen info, all clinics were running late as usual and the clinic that I wanted with Theresa was running 1 hour late so we had a long wait. My appointment had been 2.40pm. It was now 3.30pm and then I spotted Theresa. She called my name the same time as it appeared on the screen. Gaz and I entered her room and Hannah my CNS was already there waiting. It is certainly always very nice to see both Hannah or Claire my CNS team. The appointment went very well and Theresa was pleased with my ongoing response to the past Cetuximab treatment. As you know the treatment was interrupted because of my non stemi heart attack and angiogram. Theresa has decided to restart my Cetuximab treatment as it had been a successful venture in giving it to me. I will be restarting it next Monday November 10th at 11.30am. I shall await her letter to confirm what happened at this appointment and both Gaz and I left. The rest of the week went well. I was tired but otherwise not bad. My feet of course and toes are my main issue now to get sorted. It is very sore to walk so I hope it is sorted soon. My Cetuximab went ahead on Monday November 10th as planned. However, on the day My toes bled, I felt sick and my eyes bled a little from the corners. I have no idea why and it worries me a lot. For the rest of the week my bleeding continued from my toes and eyes. Sunday the 16th was a mass for my wife Joan. It's the 6th anniversary of her passing away. The day went okay.

——— # # # ———

MONDAY NOVEMBER 17th 2014 another trip to Guys to have my Cetuximab treatment. The nose bleeds are today pretty bad as is the bleeding from my toes. I hope the toe problem is sorted out soon as a priority. Nose bleeds I can handle but toes and eye bleeding is not nice. However, all my current problems that I just mentioned are certainly not enough to delay or cancel my treatment, these problems are part and parcel of having cancer and its treatment. Apart from a blood test on Thursday 20th before 11am, my problems of this bleeding continued for the entire week. My employers wanted proof that my condition was carrying a prognosis of being terminal. How sad is that when the bosses want evidence that I am going to die. Well, they got their proof. As I said all week my bleeding problems continued and a new one is cracked skin in my abdomen which is now bleeding as well. On Monday 24th my chemotherapy of Cetuximab went ahead finally on Thursday 27th I got my long awaited appointment with a Podiatrist at 9am in Orpington Hospital to hopefully set the ball rolling to sort my feet and toes out. Bit of a low time this week. I feel like the fakes who never went away are popping up again to pretend they care about me but to be honest I now know that they couldn't give a toss about me. It seems like my name cropped up and it was according to them the right time to contact me just for the sake of it and then that's done and they hide away again until their next scheduled call is due. That's not caring, that's fake caring just to keep them happy, not me.

——— # # # ———

MONDAY DECEMBER 1st, I had chemo today at 1pm, my usual Cetuximab and for some reason I feel like absolute shit after it. It is all at the wrong time as tomorrow morning my friend Lizzie from work is coming to see me and then on Thursday I travel to Razgrad in Bulgaria to see Milena. I look an absolute mess with my bleeding from face, stomach and feet. I was due a blood test to check my INR level but on Friday December 5th early morning I attended the hospital in Razgrad to have this blood test etc done. I had to pay but only a couple of quid. My INR level was 2.2 but I phoned the Warfarin Clinic in The PRUH to let them know but all was okay by them. Most of the bleeding is hidden from view apart from my face which is an absolute bloody mess. Also this week I feel abandoned by everyone. I feel that the only people who care about me now are Gaz and my sister Mary even though today, Monday DECEMBER 8th 2014, I am still in Bulgaria with Milena. There are only 17 days to Christmas and it does not feel like we are near Christmas. Obviously no chemo today as I am out here, I can honestly say that the hospital here is a shithole. It's old and filthy. I attended the hospital in Razgrad here today again and my INR was 3.2. All these readings are telephoned by me back to my Hospital in the PRUH when they then advise me to adjust my warfarin intake to prevent blood clotting. At this stage I now realise that the sooner I get home the better for my peace of mind and my personal health. Yesterday I had five separate nose bleeds and today I had three. I go home in a couple of days.

——— # # # ———

SUNDAY DECEMBER 14th 2014, I left Milena and Razgrad and made my way to Varna Airport. That was one awful journey. I need to get on that flight but I am very sick and bleeding badly. After a few hours of pain and bleeding, I got to Varna Airport and after handing over my rental car, I made my way to check in. It was very noticeable that I was in poor health and it was gradually getting worse. Of all the problems I have, it is noticeably bad bleeding from my cheek bones and people are noticeably avoiding sitting near me. Soon I will be boarding and I am now very, very nervous. Then it happened. Like a scene from a thriller movie, two security guards walked towards me. Someone had obviously complained about my condition and as I was to be on the London Luton flight with Wizz Air. I have no idea yet who complained but that person complaining were obviously concerned that I might contaminate the whole flight. Then I noticed one middle aged female who stood out a mile by paying extra attention to me and yet trying to blend in with the other passengers also waiting to board. The two security guards got nearer and soon it was obvious that I was their target. The supergrass female was nearby and watched with interest as the two security guards took me to a side room just as boarding begun. I had paid for priority boarding with Wizz Air, that was now out the window. I was in danger now of missing my flight. They asked immediately about my bleeding and I explained. I had all my paperwork and medication with me as well as my permit to fly from my doctor. That was all that was needed. After about ten minutes, they allowed me to leave their little security centre and I went straight for the boarding gate. Then I looked around me as I got on the shuttle bus out to the aircraft. On the short journey to the plane, an Airbus A320 aircraft there was no sign of the culprit woman who spilled the beans on my condition. We got to the aircraft and I climbed the front steps and got to my seat. My my, guess who is sitting in the seat in front of me? You guessed correctly, it's supergrass herself. I took my window seat. I immediately apologised for my condition to her and explained why. This was also my way of telling her that I knew she was the informant of my health condition to the security guards. She then immediately told me that she told the security that she was concerned for my health. I then told her that I knew it was her from the moment I was taken away for questioning and that it was okay. I decided that being confrontational was not good as it was a flight lasting three hours and we were stuck with each other. We took off on time and we had an enjoyable flight back to Luton apart from stemming blood loss on the way. My feet were in agony all because of my toes in both feet. However, I think I opened her eyes as to what it was like being a terminal cancer sufferer. At Luton we said goodbye and went our separate ways. I was however very relieved to be back home and it certainly made my mind up for me that soon I would be stopping my trips to Milena. My health comes first and there is a huge language barrier so it's only a matter of time before we would be breaking up for good. Long distance relationships are difficult anyway to last.

——— # # # ———

MONDAY DECEMBER 15th 2014. I am very sick. At 9.30am I went to the Warfarin Clinic and was told that my blood INR was1.3. At 1.30 in the afternoon, I went to Guys and had my Cetuximab cancer treatment. The day went okay but I felt like shit. I cannot wait to get home. After all was done and a crap train journey, I got indoors and soon went to bed. The remainder of the week went okay. Gaz and his then girlfriend came to stay on Wednesday. All week my toes continued to bleed badly but the week was interrupted with a visit to the Podiatrist in the clinic near Tescos in Orpington. Finally something is being done about these bleeding ingrowing toenails. The Podiatrist attempted to cut one of the offending bleeding nails but the actual bleeding got worse so she abandoned the procedure. On FRIDAY night DECEMBER 19th, we all went to the Christmas panto in Bromley and Gaz was here with me all weekend. Always love it when Gaz is here.

——— # # # ———

MONDAY DECEMBER 22nd 2014 Gaz was still here at home with me and would be so for the next week or so all over Christmas and New Year. Today also I had my planned usual chemo at 1.30pm. My bleeding from my body parts like toes in both feet, dry cracked cheek bones and eyes continued as before. My chemo treatment was given as usual over a few hours etc. When it was over, I made my way home by walking, train and bus. I now hide my face from the public because it is such a f*****g awful mess and there is no sign of it ending or improving. It will have to be treated with medication like Doxycycline, Aveeno Cream and Double Base Gel. Being currently in the winter months, It is pretty easy to hide my face in a wolly hat and scarf. Add to that a puffer jacket and my camouflage is complete. Now as regards the rest of the week, Gaz was still here over the Christmas and New Year period. Christmas day DECEMBER 25th was very quiet and with Gaz was great here at home but did not feel like Christmas at all. If the consultant in Guys is correct with her prognosis, then this is to be my very last Christmas alive. However, I have every intention of trying to be here next Christmas and as many of the other ones as possible.

——— # # # ———

On FRIDAY DECEMBER 26th 2014. The week ends with the bleeding etc still a major problem in my life. Lately, I tried my luck at online dating and on Sunday afternoon I was to meet a middle aged female in Stratford called A. She was Portuguese and worked as a carer in a care home. I am careful who I meet as there are so many gold diggers out there. My bleeding is bad and I explained my cancer predicament to her but she said it does not bother her at all. I wonder how much of that is actually true. I wonder if she is an exception to the rule, Lets see, eh?

——— # # # ———

MONDAY DECEMBER 29th even over this holiday period, My Chemotherapy treatment went ahead at 3.30pm. I took the train there and back and got home late in the evening.

——— # # # ———

On DECEMBER 30th and 31st, I carried home as normal but even though I also remained at home on New Years Eve 31st DECEMBER 2014 into JANUARY 1st 2015. Gaz was out as he had his own plans and it was not a problem at all. Okay It is JANUARY 1st 2015 and the start of another year fighting this f*****g horrible disease called Cancer. Right now this is one disease that has gained the upper hand. It is in fact my greatest enemy and it hates me. It hates my body and absolutely detests me as a human being. That's not all. This cancer wants me dead but it's a new year and a new start. The week was just a normal week. Same problems continued with sore bleeding toes and bleeding from my cracked skin in cheekbones and my eyes. What in the name of God puts an end to these problems.

——— # # # ———

MONDAY JANUARY 5th 2015 was a mad, mad day. In the morning on top of all my problems, I had to go to St Thomas's Hospital to have a Pet Scan at 11.15am. I got the train to Waterloo East from Orpington. I then walked up to Tommys and got there a little early for my scan. If you remember, this is the scan that takes a few hours with Radiation sugar pumped into my blood system and then after a wait of 1.5 hours, I am scanned. After all was done I then had to get a taxi to Guys as I had an appointment for Cetuximab chemo at 3.3 pm. They knew that I had a scan at 11.30am so there was a small possibility that I would be late getting to Guys for my treatment. By the end of the day I was glad to get home and indoors in the comfort of my home. I was very tired but it was down to the fact that my day was f*****g crazy busy.

——— # # # ———

On WEDNESDAY JANUARY 7th 2015. I saw Theresa, my consultant, at 11.10am to get the results of my scan that I had on Monday. Gaz was with me and my God I needed him. Theresa told me that there was a slight increase in the cancer cells in the area near the base of my tongue. The area of my neck remains under control but the tongue base is very worrying for Theresa and the team and more so for me. I was not expecting this at all and left the room in dismay. It was near as bad as my diagnosis back in 2013. I don't remember the trip home but Gaz was with me. I got indoors and chilled out as best as possible with Gaz for the rest of the evening.

——— # # # ———

THURSDAY JANUARY 8th 2015. Nice surprise. My pension paid out, enough said. The remainder of the week was quiet except for FRIDAY which required me to go to the Job Centre for 2.50pm to declare my pension pay out etc. It has to be done.

——— # # # ———

MONDAY JANUARY 12th 2015 . I attended the warfarin clinic in the PRUH to check my INR level which was 1.5 and I adjusted my warfarin intake accordingly. The remainder of the week was as follows. My bleeding problems continued. The pains and the thinking of my situation cause me so much internal anguish. I do not mention it but I cry every single night. Why in the name of God have I been selected to die at the hands of cancer. My disease is terminal and that means certain death at the hands of a disease that knows every trick in the medical books on how to wear me down and eventually put me in a position where I will need pain controlling drugs and round the clock care. I hope that I die in my sleep whenever that time comes knocking on my door. I think about death every day now. In fact, since day one all I think about is my death and what form it will take when it happens.

——— # # # ———

On THURSDAY 15th I had an appointment at 11.45am in Orpington Hospital to see a Podiatrist. I have also just met online a middle aged female but it's very early days. Apart from a warfarin clinic visit on Monday where my INR level is 2.0, I then had chemo in Guys at 11.30am.

——— # # # ———

On THURSDAY 22nd 2015 I had an appointment in the PRUH to have my Gastric band adjusted by putting fluid into it as it was previously empty and therefore no restriction. It was this way to assist in my recovery after my previous heavy doses of chemo in the past since diagnosis. The idea is no restriction means it's easier to put weight back on. Anyhow lets see. Normality resumes meaning, apart from chemo at 11.00am on MONDAY, my bleeding toe problems continue and basically it may sound boring but things start getting interesting again on MONDAY FEBRUARY 2nd 2015. It was to be a mad, mad day. Starting at 9am with a visit to the warfarin clinic in the PRUH, quickly followed by an appointment in Orpington Hospital with a visit to a podiatrist at 10.05am. The podiatrist told me that sometime in the coming weeks there would be minor surgery on my bleeding toes caused by my ingrowing toenails in both feet. To walk is just sheer agony. The podiatrist told me it would be painful as some toenails would be actually removed. As if I don't have enough pain etc in my daily life, there will be a lot in this. This was followed by a quick run to do some shopping and return home before getting the train to Guys in London for my Chemotherapy appointment at 1pm. During the remainder of the week, I was due back in Guys to see Theresa my consultant at 2.20pm but it was cancelled and on THURSDAY 5th, I was back in the PRUH seeing Starlene in her clinic, just to review my Gastric band. According to her all is very well. It was a day of cancellations as Dr G cancelled my cardiac appointment to review my heart condition. All is well anyway apart from my toes and the daily cries of loneliness and depression etc. Monday 9th the week was as follows, Chemo on the Monday at 10am in Guys followed by Tuesday 10th with a 9.15am appointment with a Podiatrist in Orpington Hospital. More chemo on MONDAY 16th at 10am and the usual problems continued. On Friday 20th there was a great boost to me when Gaz moved back home. On Monday 23rd was a Pet Scan at 11.15am in Tommys and then a dash to Guys for chemotherapy at 3.30pm.

——— # # # ———

On WEDNESDAY FEBRUARY 25th I saw Theresa my, consultant, at 3.40pm, She was alarmed with my toxicity from the Cetuximab chemo and of my bleeding in cracks in my face and toes. I told her about my planned procedures on my bleeding toenails. Theresa then told me that to give my system a rest, the infusion of Cetuximab would be stopped immediately for a period of time and that Theresa would decide when it would be resumed again. On Thursday 26th was my Warfarin clinic appointment where my INR was showing 3.7.

——— # # # ———

SUNDAY MARCH 1st was my Garreth celebrating his 25th birthday.

——— # # # ———

MONDAY 2nd MARCH my chemo was cancelled and in the warfarin clinic my INR was 1.2, a nice low figure for one reason, yes Tuesday March 3rd is my toenail surgery day. Good morning, it's surgery day and I am in Beckenham Beacon Hospital where my toenail operation begins soon this morning. I have been told to expect absolutely awful, sometimes unbearable, pain. I will write again afterwards as my toenail Beckenham Butcher has arrived and I am first on his list to go under the knife. Hi again, three hours ago I was lying down and it started. Sharp scratch must be the biggest f*****g lie said by any person with a needle and intending to stick it somewhere. It was awful as he injected each of the 8 toes facing the chop. His needles injecting local anaesthetic went into the bones in all of the toes facing nail removal or alteration. I screamed in pain as I felt those needles going in and as soon as they emptied their numbing liquid contents, I knew those needles were inside each toe right up against the toe bones. Big toes or small toes, they all got the same amount of numbing liquid and same size needles. Can you imagine what it looked like, and I watched it all as the numbing was only local. The worst part was watching the nail being cut away and lifted off the toe and all the glistening red blood just left. I only felt pulling and tugging as he pulled on each of the nails. The pain relief and anaesthetic was wearing off. I heard those magic words. Sharp scratch. After near three hours later it was all over and he wrapped each of the toes individually. All over with 4 nails gone and 4 trimmed and partially removed. I made one blunder, no slippers with me. In fact no other footwear apart from the shoes I brought with me and they would not be worn by me again for many weeks to come. The surgeon gave me some blue plastic bags to put on my feet. I left and contacted a cab firm to pick me up and take me home. It could only happen to me. I got a take away cup of coffee and waited outside the hospital front main entrance. As I stood there with paper cup in hand and no shoes just two blue plastic foot covers and bandaged toes, a middle aged woman going in assumed I was homeless and begging and took out her purse to give me some money. I explained to her that I just had surgery and my toes were just bandaged and covered up. We both laughed but I knew that my laugh would be shortlived because of my pain in each of my eight damaged twinkletoes. I think she knew that as well. As soon as she turned her back and walked away, my smile stopped. I did not find it funny, but was only being polite. My cab arrived and I went home. I spent the remainder of the day just resting, feet up for the rest of the day. I was certainly glad today was over. Now I need them to heal over the coming weeks.

——— # # # ———

On WEDNESDAY MARCH 4TH 2015 I had an appointment at 11am with Dr Garbi my cardiologist. All went well and some medication was stopped as my heart was good now.

——— # # # ———

On FRIDAY 6th was a blood test at 10.30am followed by my Podiatrist in Orpington checking on my eight twinkletoes. She was happy with the healing process of all eight toes.

——— # # # ———

MONDAY MARCH 9th 2015. No chemo treatment today. Because of my toxic reaction to it, the break from Cetuximab continues. I had a blood test at 10.30am and my INR was checked.

——— # # # ———

On WEDNESDAY 11th, I met Theresa in her clinic at 10.30am and as my toxicity was still very obvious, further time was given by her for me to recover but also that a trial drug involving a placebo was coming on the scene soon. A placebo, you may know, means I may get a simple sweet or innocent capsule or tablet. I would never know if I got the real thing or not. Right now I will take anything that gives me a chance at extending my life. My torment continues however.

——— # # # ———

On FRIDAY 13th 2015 I had another INR test and it read 2.2. so far so good. Also the same day at 1.30pm, I had an appointment with my podiatrist to check

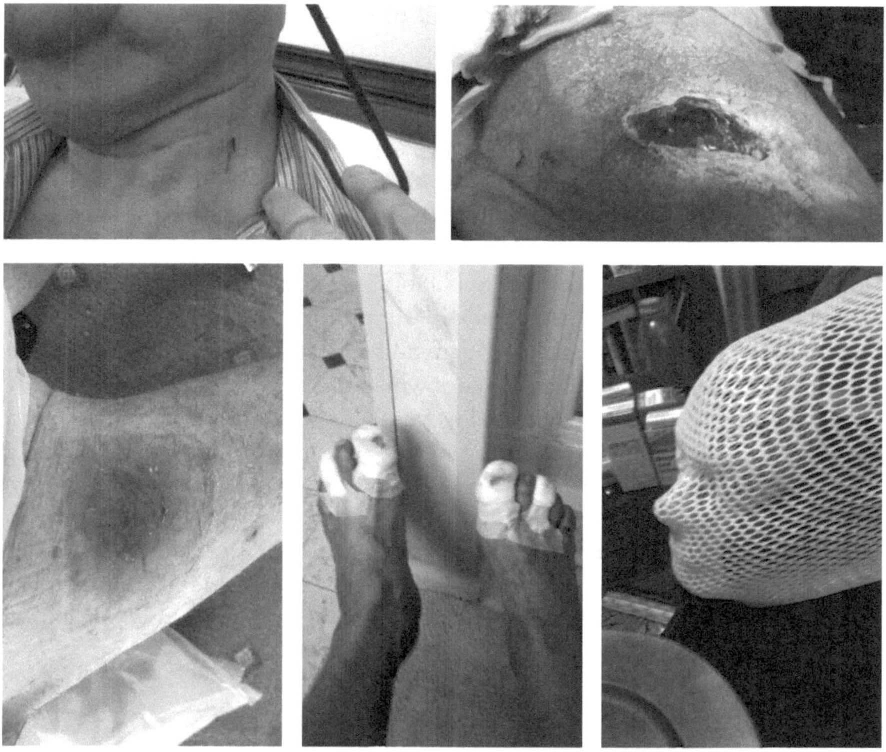

The effects cancer treatment has on your feet and body.

on my toes, those with and without nails. The following week all progressed as normal. No more bleeding from toes and face etc. Just shows what chemotherapy can do to the body. The only excitement this week was on Tuesday 17th with a reading INR of 3.2, this was high and my warfarin was altered to reduce the reading. The other excitement was a trip to see my podiatrist on Friday 20th. The following week had Monday 23rd an INR reading of 3.6, Thursday 26th my gastric band had 9.5 mls of fluid put in it to restrict it even more and more excitement on Friday with INR reading 2.8. This was followed at 2.20pm by another visit to the podiatrist in Orpington. The following week on TUESDAY 31st MARCH 2015 at 9am had an INR reading of 4.0. At 11.20am my podiatrist checked my toes and re dressed them. She was very pleased with the healing and so was I.

——— # # # ———

WEDNESDAY APRIL 1st 2015, I met my consultant at 9.30am and we discussed my starting on a trial named BERYL trial and a CT scan would be organised to have prior to me starting this trial, followed at 10am by a MUGA SCAN. The bleeding on my toes has now almost completely gone. Now more exciting news. For the past year my son and I were almost certainly deciding to have a conservatory at the rear of our home. Anglian windows were the ones we chose to build it and on Monday April 6th 2018 we agreed a price. My real reason for having a conservatory was so that I would have somewhere to rest and relax after undergoing treatment and also to add value to my home. I have always wanted a conservatory and now I am about to have one and spend my time recovering from my treatment. The original cost of the conservatory was £29,000 but as I agreed to pay it back in 10 months, it only cost me £16,000. Tuesday 7th I had INR check at 8.30am and at 10.05am a podiatrist check in Orpington Hospital to look at my toes which are now healing very well. My chemotherapy still has not restarted as yet. This was all repeated on 14th in warfarin clinic with an INR reading of 4.0 and at 11.45am a podiatrist. To recap now on my current problems are as follows. Toes recovering from surgery, tiredness, bleeding from sores on my face especially my cracked skin on cheekbones, very sporadic INR blood levels with high and low readings and difficult to get correct level of warfarin tablets. My chemotherapy treatment has been temporarily suspended until my bleeding and facial cuts and sores have begun to clear up.

——— # # # ———

On FRIDAY APRIL 17th 2015, I attended the warfarin clinic without an appointment as I had a terrible nose bleed in the morning. I went there at 2.30pm and on being checked it soon showed that I had an INR reading of 5.1. This was the highest yet and showed that my blood was so thinned out now, it was like water in my veins. Is it no wonder that I bled and bled so much. At 4.20pm another doctor came to see me and this followed with a visit to my GP.

——— # # # ———

On MONDAY APRIL 20th my INR check showed a remarkable drop to an acceptable level of 1.9. At 2.30pm was a visit from Anglian homes surveyor to set the ball rolling to build my conservatory. Tuesday 21st at 10.30pm was a trip to see my podiatrist in Orpington Hospital. She was happy with my toes and I dare say that my toes were over the moon to see her. At 2.15pm was a trip to Guys to have a CT scan on my head, neck and body. On Wednesday 22nd, I saw Theresa my consultant who gave me the bad news that I was not accepted on the trial drug list because of my previous heart condition. I am annoyed and upset as I had that CT scan yesterday on 21st and a day later today the trial drug people rejected me. The recent PET SCAN showed an increase of my cancer, so treatment of some kind must happen soon. I am now being considered for treatment by more chemotherapy of Carboplatin and Paclitaxel. I left the room both disappointed and yet hopeful about the new chemotherapy being planned for me. Thursday 23rd was in the Warfarin clinic with an INR reading of only 1.4, a good reading. To show you how sporadic my INR blood readings are, only a few days ago was 1.4, well today Monday 27th at 9am in the same warfarin clinic was 2.5. How mad is that?

——— # # # ———

TUESDAY 28th APRIL at 1.55pm was a podiatrist visit in Orpington Hospital.

——— # # # ———

WEDNESDAY APRIL 29th 2015 at 1.30pm, I had an appointment with Theresa or Andriana of the same team. My toxicity has improved somewhat and Theresa agreed to hold off any treatment for now and after a Pet Scan in two months, any treatment may be based on that. Apart from an INR reading on April 30th which showed a 2.4 there is nothing exciting really to report. Tuesday May 5th a podiatrist reviewed my post surgery toes. All is well on that part of the body. I had a very bad nose bleed on Thursday 7th and I went to the warfarin clinic. This is now getting repeated stuff, so very soon I will stop writing my weekly or twice weekly visits and the readings. I knew the reading was high and it was 4.3. My nose bleeds continued pretty bad for the next few days.

——— # # # ———

On SATURDAY MAY 9th 2015, my sister who still calls me every day, arrived from home in Ireland with my niece Aishling to see me. Nice surprise. The nose bleeds carried on as bad as ever. Mary and Aishling went back home on Monday 11th and afterwards on that afternoon a trip to the warfarin clinic showed a reading of 4.3. Still too high so it's no wonder that I am bleeding a lot from my nose. The nose bleeds continued all week and to be honest I am now fed up of that f*****g warfarin clinic. Thursday had a reading of 3.7. On Monday 18th, my INR was 3.0 and that's it. My warfarin clinic trips were every week for the forseeable future with no sign of it ending. My podiatrist saw me on 19th and soon I expect these appointments to be less frequent as the healing of my toes improves. When my visits come to an end then I will write here to tell you. Until then you can take it that all these frequent appointments on toes and INR continue. On May 26th building work on my conservatory began.

——— # # # ———

On JUNE 24th 2015 at 10.30am, I had a Pet Scan in St Thomas's hospital. This is important as it will give an up-to-date true reading of what the cancer is doing to me, especially as I have had no treatment in ages. In a way I am worried about the end result as I have conditioned myself to be dependent on chemo etc. The building of my conservatory progressed well, so well that I am now getting the flooring down and finishing touches on the whole structure. My health was good, very few nose bleeds and as a result I met someone online called Marie. On the 6th we went to Elstree to a recording of Pointless TV show but failed to get in. It was a good omen as that person soon fizzled out of my life.

——— # # # ———

On WEDNESDAY JULY 8th at 12 noon I met Theresa in Oncology. We discussed the scan as it showed a slight increase in cancer at the base of the tongue area. I feel good and overall she is happy with me. She is going to request a Pet Scan again in 3 months as a surveillance scan and in the meantime she and the team will look further on this scan result. Gaz, who was with me as he always is for these meetings, was very relieved as I was. We left her room content and relieved.

——— # # # ———

On THURSDAY JULY 17th, a person who I thought was a good friend of mine proved that she was a complete and utter f*****g fake. She promised this and that and I did suspect something and was on my guard. No, she got no money but her stories were just all lies, lies and lies. I will not name her but you would think that someone who works in the health business would be okay. No she was not, lying bitch, but I noticed it early and my judgement was correct.

——— # # # ———

On MONDAY JULY 27th my podiatrist saw me at the clinic near Tescos in Orpington. She was so pleased with my toe recovery that I am not due back for 6 months from now. The warfarin clinic however continues to see me on a very regular basis so we carry on with it as before. Thursday August 6th was the 1st anniversary of Gaz and his girlfriend. I love them both so much. Okay, my storyline begins to get exciting and full of controversy very soon. The name to make a note of is Mr J, a very good consultant and my life would soon change for the better and … well, let me just say that it would be a long time before I believe people any more and what they promise. My appointment with him was 2.45pm but was not seen until 3.20pm on THURSDAY AUGUST 13th 2015. He told me amazing news. He said he had looked closer at my last PET Scan and he was able to set a date to operate on the cancer in my throat. It was really amazing news and it boosted me so much. I wanted to tell the world that back in 2013/14 they told me that I had 18 months to live and now this man was going to promise me the world and an end to my cancer and an amazing future. Gaz was not with me today so he was the first that I phoned. Everyone that I spoke to were over the moon about my news. I am in shock and a little not expecting to hear so lets see. I don't remember leaving his room, I don't remember the journey home or even reaching home. The next day was Friday and on that day and all over weekend I still cannot believe what this man has promised me.

——— # # # ———

On THURSDAY 20TH AUGUST 2015 I was in the PRUH to have my band adjusted and emptied of all fluid prior to my throat surgery. This meeting in the PRUH was organised at very short notice.

——— # # # ———

On TUESDAY AUGUST 25th I again saw Mr J about my surgery at 2.30pm. He said that I was not a candidate at this stage for Immunotherapy. He has told me that the surgery will happen on Monday September 7th. In the meantime, I feel good and no issues at all. Could it really all be happening for me at last? Were all the prayers being answered? Was I really going to be getting rid of my cancer finally? I feel good, maybe just maybe. On Sunday September 6th, I went into Guys with the intention of preparing myself for surgery on my throat and Mr J was to remove my cancerous tumour and effectively give me my life back. I had stopped taking my warfarin so bleeding risk was removed for the operation to go ahead.

——— # # # ———

Today, at 9am SEPTEMBER 7th 2015, I was taken into theatre and before long I was asleep. A couple of hours later I think, I woke up in recovery all done. It was a quick recovery and that night, at 9pm, I was on my way home having been discharged correctly. I still cannot believe it. I have no pain as I am having a lot of morphine but am sure that will soon wear off. However, on Wednesday 9th the morphine was wearing off and I am now in pain, which is gradually increasing. I am also lonely as Gaz went to Hong Kong last night for a few weeks to work. I am going to miss him but it's work and it has to be done. Thursday 10th I am crying. It's a time of mixed emotions. Gaz is away and I am trying to cope with the fact that Mr J has promised my life back and I so, so want to believe him. On Saturday September 12th, I attended my Street Party in my road. It was great organising it and gave me a purpose in life to aim for. The day went great and even though I was in pain, I thoroughly enjoyed it. Over the following few days, my throat etc was very painful and I cannot eat via my mouth. I still cry at what happened me back in 2013 and what is currently going on. I am enjoying the summer despite my state of health and mind. I am also worried about Friday. I will see Mr J and find out if all that he has promised is actually true.

——— # # # ———

FRIDAY SEPTEMBER 18th 2015, I saw Mr J in Guys at 12 noon. I cried and cried on the way. I saw him and he told me that they went in via my mouth during the surgery and he removed the cancer tumour area etc. He also told me that they got it all and that they also removed some good tissue so as to ensure that they got all the cancer. Mr J then said, congratulations, you got your life back, enjoy it all. He then shook my hand and I left his consultation room. It was fantastic news but too often I have been let down and I am in mixed thoughts right now. All I can say to Mr J is, … "thank you for what you done by giving me my life back". I got home and told Gaz even though he is in Hong Kong. I told so many people, family first, then friends. Everyone is so happy for my news, but, what if there is going to be a spanner in the works. Right now, I am enjoying life. On Saturday 19th my brother Liam arrived to see me. It's nice to see him so he can see what state I am in. I think he finds it difficult to accept my cancer and that I will probably die from it. He is my brother and I love him so, so much. On Monday September 21st a strange thing came over me and I feel so depressed and lonely. My good news about my surgery means nothing today. I feel lost, lonely, depressed and nothing like someone who has been promised my life back and cancer gone. Is my body telling me that the cancer is not gone? On today Friday 25th, I got a letter in post from Mr J that I am clear of cancer, Yet am I really clear of the big C? The letter also stated that a new scan is to be ordered for 4 weeks time. It seems very soon but maybe they know best. My loneliness is still present with no sign of it going away. On Tuesday 29th I was down for a pet scan booked a long time ago but Mr J or H the secretary cancelled it. I still feel lonely and depressed. On Thursday October 1st, I met my partner during online dating. I feel boosted and not too depressed. Let us see how this is going to go. Gaz is happy for me. On October 3rd Gaz arrived back from Hong Kong. My health is not bad but my feet are both numb today, no explanation for this. Tuesday 6th both feet and many fingers feel numb.

——— # # # ———

Today is OCTOBER 7th 2015 and it's my 58th birthday. This is one birthday that I was not meant to be celebrating. I should have died a long time ago from this vicious cancer. Somehow, and I do not know why, but am still here. I am now aiming to start feeling better and maybe having Miss S will do me some good … I hope so, please God. My partner and I went out to a restaurant in Bexley for my birthday. Is this all too good to be true?

——— # # # ———

OCTOBER 8th THURSDAY 2015. This morning I have neck spasm and both feet and fingers are numb. What next, I wonder, is going to come my way. It carried on for a number of days but there is no reason for it apart from the treatment up to now. I am also relieved to be able to say that my throat pain from the surgery is now a lot beter and it is getting easier to eat and swallow a little more now. All soft food for now as the gastric band is due for further tightening soon. On Monday October 12th I had an appointment with my cardiologist at 4pm to have an Echo test on my heart. My numbness etc in feet and fingers is Peripheral neurapathy. It is a condition that I have to put up with for a long time to come and yes it is because of treatment up to now. My partner and I are doing okay. On Wednesday 14th there was a phone call from Theresa my consultant just to see how I was coping since my good news. She said a Pet Scan would be arranged soon to monitor everything. My new ailments now are numbness and tingling which is Peripheral neurapathy and random neck rash. On Friday 16th my GP Dr Nicholls saw me in his surgery and was just to tell me that he was happy with my echo test results. He also gave me a flu jab. On Monday 19th, Dr Garbi also gave me clearance to fly. Fly where you may ask? Gaz is in Hong Kong and is due back so I have decided, while I am reasonably well, that I will go to Hong Kong for a week and then Gaz and I come back home together. I am so looking forward to it but I am going out there alone. Miss S is not coming with me. I need time alone with Gaz anyway and this is my big chance. On Thursday night November 5th, I flew to Hong Kong. I had an amazing week there, various restaurants every night, Korean, Mongolian, Chinese. I did everything in Hong Kong. I took the Ferry to Hong Kong Island and took a bus down to Stanley beach where the Japanese butchered the Chinese during the occupation. Overall, I had the best week ever. I took the underground out to Li Chi Nunnery and saw the 10,000 buddhas which was amazing an spectacle. Other restaurants Gaz and I went to were Mexican, Nepalese and Taiwanese. On Friday 13th Gaz and I flew back from Hong Kong. The flights there and return were on the Virgin Dreamliner. That too was amazing. On the Saturday morning after we landed in Heathrow, my leg went from under me and I was taken off the plane in a wheelchair. It got better enough for me to drive home. I went to A and E that evening to be told that I needed a new knee. What next for me? I went to mass on Sunday as it was an anniversary mass for my late wife Joan. It has been 7 years now since she passed away on November 16th 2008 but it feels like yesterday. I saw my partner on and off here in my place but for some reason she never invited me into her house. On Thursday November 19th, my gastric band was checked by Starr in the PRUH in her clinic. All is well there. My peripheral problems etc continue.

——— # # # ———

On SATURDAY NOVEMBER 28th 2015, I was coughing up blood. It carried on the next day as well. Okay, now it's time to tell you a true story about an ex neighbour of mine who lived near me at a previous address. I will not name him but this is one funny story that I have to share with you. Right, here we go. A number of years ago at a previous address I had two neighbours who were brothers and they moved to Suffolk. We kept in contact however and every year we got a Christmas card from them and of course we sent them a card. We also spoke on the phone now and again and of course last year I told one of them that I had terminal cancer. Okay so far so good but this morning I had one of those phone calls. When I answered the phone, the brother that I spoke to said to me "Garreth"? I said no. "It's Dave here". His reply was priceless. He simply said "Shouldn't you be dead". This was followed by "We were doing the cards and we thought we should check to see if you had passed away before we write and send you a Christmas card". I assured him I was alive and he then said he would post me a card tomorrow. I then thought to myself, that's it, he would not waste a card, envelope, ink and a stamp on me just in case I had died, so he had to check first. Is that what I am worth in some peoples minds? And then I thought, I just have to laugh it off so I decided to ring him now every November if I am still alive and just to guarantee at least one Christmas card. So it's funny how some people sort out their priorities different to most normal people. I wonder, will they be shocked when I call them next time? I dare not forget or they will be turning up with flowers to my funeral. So you know know that this book has humorous parts in it as well as sad and tearful sections.

——— # # # ———

MONDAY DECEMBER 7th 2015. A Pet Scan was due today but someone in Oncology, either a secretary or appointments, has seriously messed up and cancelled my Pet Scan due today or around now. Mr J had operated and said he got all the cancer and to make sure that they got it all, said that they got some healthy tissue too. However, I cannot believe him until I have this scan and now that's not happening. I complained to Theresa today and told her and was told that the slots were full but a scan would be organised as soon as possible. I hope so as it is the only true way of finding out if Mr J actually gave me a cancer free future. He has built my hopes up so much – what do I do if he is wrong. Now I am crying thinking about it all. This should be the happiest time of my life but it's not.

——— # # # ———

FRIDAY DECEMBER 11th 2015. Went to the Churchill Theatre for the Christmas Panto. So many friends and ex work colleagues and their families went with me. My partner went with me and she met everyone on the night. I was tired but enjoyed going out. It has been ages since I had a good night out. Over the next few days my lymph nodes in my neck area were very swollen. My throat is also very sore. Now I am even more worried and as yet no sign of a scan being organised. On Monday morning 14th December, I again called Oncology and simply begged for a Pet Scan. On Thursday December 17th was an appointment in the PRUH to adjust my gastric band. Nine mls of fluid was put into it, to give it some restriction. Christmas is only around the corner but I didn't let my cancer get in my way. I managed my Christmas shopping as normal and gave away Christmas presents, as I always do. I still have lumps in my throat and they are sore, however it now looks like I can eat very little over Christmas. I am now convinced that Mr J did not get all my cancer and my remission is short lived as I am convinced my cancer is back with a vengeance. All over Christmas and New year I was only able to eat very little but my lumps and soreness are now all very obvious and very, very sore. I pray that I have a Pet Scan very very soon and yet sometimes I pray that it will end quickly and I have a painless death. If my cancer has returned, there is nothing treating it and I am very, very anxious. I also have a new problem with cramps in my feet now added to the list of my current problems.

——— # # # ———

DECEMBER 31st NEW YEARS EVE 2015. My partner was at home with her grown up kids and I was at home alone, seeing in new year. I didn't mind as I had time to think about things, my cancer and my future. What future in 2016 do I actually have?

——— # # # ———

FRIDAY JANUARY 1st 2016. Can I wish everyone a very Happy New Year 2016. I have no idea if this year will be good for me or not. However, as for my future, I hope it's a good one. I say this every year because the previous year has in all cases been shit. I can in all honesty say that 2013 was okay until the diagnosis of my terminal cancer towards the end of that year made sure of a shit year. In 2014 the chemotherapy and what it done to my body and mind certainly guaranteed that it too was a shit year. What can I say about then, the year just passed being 2015. It was basically my body suffering inside and outside. My body has suffered terribly with much of it to the point of never ever recovering physically and even sometimes mentally. It is also because of bits of treatment on and off being tried and tested and then stopped. Now you know why they are in my mind nothing but shit years and here we are in 2016 and it is certainly looking like a repeat of the previous years and treatments and facing more prolonged agony again. As it is January 1st 2016, today my partner and her family are here for lunch and getting to meet me and my Gaz . I did the cooking where I made my own favourite, a lasagne. I have peripheral neurapathy with also suffering cramps in my legs My right knee is very sore and apart from having some lumps in my neck outside. Inside also is me having a very sore inside throat. The same problems continued all week and reached a nasty time on Thursday 7th January 2016 when I started coughing up blood. I am now convinced that Mr J has got it all wrong and I am near certain that my cancer is back. I am now begging for a scan, a Pet Scan. I want that scan now. As well as that my trips to the warfarin clinic continue with crazy mixed readings as before. I will refer to it now and again as before. I am also phoning my consultant every few days asking for that Pet Scan. Every day now I am spitting up blood which is very worrying. Previously I was told any changes or bleeding etc to tell them. Well I tell them but no sign of a scan happening. Why, why, why? Wednesday, January 20th 2016, today is my partner's birthday and same problems and today also a nose bleed is back. I have also today received a letter to attend the clinic of Mr J in Guys on Friday 22nd January 2016.

——— # # # ———

Hi all, fast forward to January 22nd and my visit to Mr J. On the way up to Guys by train, I was terrified. No scan but why does he want to see me. Everything is now going through my mind. I cannot even remember if I spoke to Peter at Orpington Station. He is normally on one of the platforms. On the train journey up to London Bridge, I cannot remember anything. The trip up to London was vacant in my mind and yet I knew I was terrified of meeting Mr J. When I got there to his clinic, I spotted him after waiting about 20 minutes. Then I was called to a room. It was not the room of Mr J but that of another member of his team. Why was Mr J avoiding me. Everything was going through my mind. The other doctor that saw me then asked if he could put a camera down my throat. The result was devastating to me as he then removed the camera and looked me straight in my eye and said "Mr Cosgrave, I am sorry but it appears to be looking like a lump in there at the place where the surgery was but we need a scan to be sure." I knew it, my f*****g cancer had come back and all along I was right. He also said that Radiotherapy was a possibility if it was the case that the cancer had come back. I left that room and now I know why Mr J was avoiding me today, or am I making a mistake with that. I hate that man right now after what he has done to me. What annoys me most is that Mr J put it in writing that I was cancer free and I put it in a frame at home, now look at my situation. If I had been given a scan when I was asking them late last year for one, maybe they would have got it earlier. They have made a huge medical blunder and my life is now under threat again. On Saturday 23rd Gaz and I had a chat about what has now happened again and what a mistake by Mr J. I am convinced that Mr J is ruthless and all he wants is self glorification. I am also back to daily and nightly crying again. I don't want to die but right now Mr J has renewed my death sentence and as a direct result guaranteed my crying every day and night. I hate him so much. He can go to his private clinic in Switzerland or his plush house or whatever while I sit here crying after he has sent me to die. Theresa is who I need now. She always gives me good news but Mr J is like my own personal private grim reaper. I am scared, scared, scared.

——— # # # ———

WEDNESDAY JANUARY 27th 2016. Today is the day of that urgent Pet Scan to see if my cancer has come back. I think it has, the recent camera down throat saw a lump so now it's the Pet Scan in St Thomas's at 1.45 pm. Mary, my sister, is coming tonight as tomorrow night I have tickets to see Graham Norton recording his show in London near Waterloo Station in The London Studios. My peripheral neurapathy. As regards the scan, I am alone for it and am terrified. Friday JANUARY 29th 2016, today at 11.30am is a big day. I have an appointment to so see that man Mr J. He confirmed that my cancer is back and there is a tumour of 4 mms in the same place that he operated on late last year. What a prick to f*** my life up like that. He said that he will refer me back to Theresa my consultant to see if Radiotherapy is an option to reduce in size or destroy that tumour. He messed up and now he is running away. One good thing is that Theresa is back on my side helping me. Mr J can run but I will be keeping my eye out for him. I feel lonely and now wondering what my death will be like. I now have to put the envelope about my funeral details and organising it back in order. In it will be my wishes when the time comes so that it will be easier for Gaz to organise. I dread what I am facing and if that envelope was ready now, I would seriously want to die right now to make it quick. Tuesday February 2nd 2016, I feel different today. I now want to fight this cancer but if this planned Radiotherapy fails then I may die this year some time.

——— # # # ———

WEDNESDAY FEBRUARY 3rd 2016. I met Theresa my consultant today at 2pm and Bless her, she confirmed that I would begin my Radiotherapy soon for 5 weeks of intensive treatment, that's every day for 5 weeks Monday to Friday. The Radiotherapy should begin in around 3 weeks from now. I trust Theresa a lot.

——— # # # ———

FRIDAY FEBRUARY 5th 2016. I received a letter in post from that guy Mr J apologising for a misprint. He said to me in his letter that he got all the cancer and that he did tell me that as it was all based on a diagnosis he made to me when he diagnosed me first in 2015. LIES. He was never the one to diagnose me as it was Theresa who diagnosed me way back in 2013. He also said that his stating that he got all the cancer was a misprint. LIES.... what he put in print, I have it framed. Why does he feel that he has to lie to me so much? Anyway, I never encountered Mr J until late 2015 when Theresa passed me over to him. He is making himself out to be a big boy. I could take it further but I may need all these medical people one day. For now I chose to take no further action as I am back in Theresa's hands and, as far as I am concerned, her hands are safe for me. Keep J, that ruthless butcher away from me! My problems now are as follows: sore throat which is also a lump, sore right knee, Peripheral neurapathy and a lot of mouth sores and blisters. As part of the planning for my upcoming Radiotherapy, I have an appointment today, Tuesday February 8th 2016, here in St Thomas's to get fitted with a mould of a mask of my facial shape. At 10am I have this fitting. This mask when completed fits over my face and I am bolted on to the table during the treatment when it does begin. Anyhow, I also have a CT scan this morning at 11.10am, also here in St Thomas's. On Thursday February 11th 2016, I went to Esther ward in Guys to discuss the possibility in future to have a nasal feed tube fitted at some stage in near future. They also told me that this feed tube may at one stage be inserted into my belly and therefore directly into stomach via abdominal wall. I was told to expect 30 sessions of Radiotherapy at a maximum dose. For some reason I had expected 5 weeks or 25 sessions. I also made it clear that I am making a formal complaint about Mr J. As well as all the current problems, I now have blisters and sores on my lips. I actually look a right mess. When I start Radiotherapy can you imagine what that is going to do to me. I have now also been given a list of dates of the Radiotherapy treatments. I have also requested a list of all treatments that I had since day one. I do not trust J at all and as yet he has not replied to me about my complaint. However, I have been told that I am to see him on March 1st 2016 at 12.15 in the afternoon. Back to today where I saw a podiatrist in Orpington at the clinic near Tesco. All is well and was told to come back in 6 months from now. Also today at 1.50pm my gastric band was checked and has 9.5 mls of fluid in it. My weight is 89. 8 kilos. Also, as yet still no reply from J so I am now looking forward to our meeting on March 1st 2016. My problems are now increasing especially where I now have a lot of difficulty in swallowing and all this just days before my Radiotherapy begins. I can now feel that awful lump in my throat. It is big and it is very sore now. In a way I cannot wait for Radiotherapy to start and in another way I am terrified of it actually beginning. I hate J for putting me in this position.

——— # # # ———

TUESDAY FEBRUARY 23rd 2016. Today is Day 1 of my Radiotherapy. It was meant to be yesterday but one of the machines broke down. Anyhow here we are and I will try to explain to you in as much detail as possible. My God. How am I going to do 30 days of this. OK, here we go. I got to Guys Hospital and followed the signs to Radiotherapy Department in the Basement of the hospital. I was terrified on the journey up there on the train. I have no idea what is facing me, no idea at all. Okay, I read all the leaflets, googled it and looked on You Tube about the machines used etc., and it may all be good and helpful but nothing prepares you for the real event. This is my personal event about to start so here we go. Sorry, I side tracked. Here we are in the Basement of Guys Hospital in the Radiotherapy. We are in the basement, the pits or the bowels of this great hospital and being here means that it is mainly hidden from the main part of the hospital. The clinical and ordinary waste is carried through this area to be eventually disposed. There is a strange smell here, a clinical smell. Anyhow the lift doors opened as we reached the basement. I stepped out and it is nothing like the floors above. Down here is like a time lapse and almost opposite the lift is the door with entry to a corridor leading to the Radiotherapy Department. I went through the doors and around the corner and got to the Radiotherapy Dept. Up to now, in the lift, in the basement, into the corridor leading here, was no sign of another human being. As soon as I got in through those doors, a new place full of life opened up in front of me. There were people, patients waiting, nurses and Radiotherapy staff. There was even a receptionist. This was a whole new place of living people that one does not expect in a place down her, with no apparent sign of life from the outside. I gave in my appointment card and simply waited my turn to be called. I put on a gown and went through to the next place to wait. I was called and then led into a room. All these rooms are called ELECTRA 5 or 6. Each room has a raised long table like bench. Today I was in ELECTRA 6 and I lay down on the bench. The mask that was already prepared for me earlier was placed over my face as I lay down but was facing upwards. I could feel this mask tighten as I was then having the head and shoulders areas bolted tightly and secured to the bench. I could not move. My hands were secured and if I now had an itch then it was tough shit. I then heard the machine come to life and for the next ten minutes or so the treatment was given to me or should I say zapped into me. I had already had a tattoo spot in the centre of my chest which is there for life. It basically indicates the exact centre of my chest etc for the benefit of the radiotherapy machine etc. I was in that room on my own but was monitored at all times. I was however, absolutely terrified as I was physically unable to move and it felt claustrophobic. It also was my first time and all the Googling and You Tube videos will never prepare you for this terrifying experience. I say terrifying because for me it was terrifying as it was new and I didn't know what to expect. When the machine stopped and its noise eased down I knew it was over, but only for today. I was facing another 29 sessions like this and the damage that it would do to me made me wonder if it was all worth it. I had my doubts all over again. All the fears came back. I was terrified of what the future would have in store for me. The things that I had been told about Radiotherapy and what it does to the human body varied. My treatment is directly on the side of my neck aimed at my base of tongue where the tumour is. Of course, whatever is in the way also gets hit by the Radiotherapy at the same time. So thirty sessions all aimed at the exact same area is bound to cause very nasty side effects. Today however all I want to do is get out of here and get home and it can't come quick enough. I left the area after getting dressed and collected my appointment card for tomorrow and a repeat performance by both them and I. I didn't feel any different as I left the area and as I was in the corridor leading from the Radiotherapy Dept I noticed that this smell from earlier was only in this corridor and seemed to ease off in severity before I got into the basement area outside the lift. I suppose it's a smell associated with this part of the basement. I got into a lift and was whisked straight to the upper floor which was the ground floor. On reaching there, the door opened and I stepped out into fresh air. I left the hospital and made my way to the train station and eventually home to my own comfortable surroundings. I checked my post and as yet no reply from Mr J. There was one letter however and it was a list of all my visits, scans and various treatments from way back in the early days when diagnosed first in 2013. Mr J had better not lie now as I had it in black and white and it was only recently that he came in contact with me with his big idea to remove my tumour etc etc and we know where that went. I am now also needing Difflam Spray on my throat to ease and numb the pain in the back of my throat. J had really caused my problems to increase now. This evening I also put it in my Facebook page that I am going to write this book about my journey with this horrible cancer. I just took it easy for the remainder of the evening and went through my experience of the day.

——— # # # ———

WEDNESDAY FEBRUARY 24th 2016 was another day in Radiotherapy. Today I would be in ELECTRA 5 at 2.50pm. For the rest of the week Miss S was with me while I had the treatments in the various rooms. By the Friday

26th. I could realise that this treatment was going to hurt me even more and cause many further problems. I feel so rough now because of this Radiotherapy and am beginning to hate this treatment. The Radiotherapy treatment however progressed with a break from it on February 28th for one day. The next day, treatment once again resumed with the consequences causing me terrible problems and suffering. Peripheral Neurapathy was terrible as was feeling sick and terrible red raw inside my throat. It is sore all the time already with blisters and ulcers some of which are now bleeding occasionally and to think that today was only Day 6 out of the 30 planned for me.

——— # # # ———

WEDNESDAY MARCH 2nd was a busy day with Blood test and INR in the morning in the PRUH, followed by catching a train to Guys to see my Consultant at 4pm and Radiotherapy in Electra 5 at 6pm. I could not wait to get home and settle down for the evening or what was left of it. Thursday was as bad with a 4pm appointment in Speech and Language in Guys followed by Radiotherapy at 6pm in Electra 5. The smell is still in the corridor of the Radiotherapy Dept, in case anybody is curious. Friday March 4th I had a blood transfusion at 1pm and at 5.15pm, I had Radiotherapy in Electra 6. My body condition is now getting worse on a day-to-day basis because of this Radiotherapy. I now have blisters and sores on my lips, ulcers on my cheek bones and now the taste takes hold and burns me from the inside out. In my mouth is the taste again, as a metallic type which I had previously in Chemo, so did not expect it with Radiotherapy. My jaw is also stiff and my skin being bad means that I now cannot shave as I bleed easily. I am also now developing a hatred or disgust of healthy people. Why should they be allowed to be healthy and smiling and enjoying life while I am suffering, looking very sick and basically feeling like I am not just waiting to die but now I simply just want to die. I am sorry but I am so low tonight now.

——— # # # ———

MARCH 5th and 6th no treatment.

——— # # # ———

MARCH 7th MONDAY, back in Guys for blood test at 4pm followed at 5pm in Electra 6 with Radiotherapy. Now also, I have coughs and sniffles also now with my sores and ulcers in eyes and face. Of course, my peripheral problems are also very obvious.

——— # # # ———

TUESDAY MARCH 8th is day 12 of radiotherapy and it's in Electra 6 at 12.30pm. This was followed by other days after my meeting my consultant on Wednesday March 9th where she increased the pain killers and especially the morphine.

——— # # # ———

THURSDAY MARCH 10th 2016 the metallic taste which has been very noticeable in recent days is now very prominent. To think that only very recent things were so much better than what they are now. Now is an absolute f*****g mess, just look at what this radiotherapy is doing to me and day-by-day it's getting worse. Sixteen sessions left and I am so messed up inside and outside. I dread what's ahead for me. As I already said, I hate healthy people at the moment, I hate the healthy people who help me medically. I detest therefore the people who make mistakes and get away with it. I also got a message today on my house phone that a blood transfusion is planned for me on Monday 14th. My radiotherapy progressed however on a daily basis.

——— # # # ———

SATURDAY MARCH 12th, My good friend Foteini and her mum came to see me today. I am now getting body shocks like a bolt of electricity going through my body.

——— # # # ———

MONDAY MARCH 14th 2016 in Guys my blood test was at 9am where it was cross matched prior to transfusion. At 9.40am was Radiotherapy in Electra 5. This was followed at 10.30am by the blood transfusion of 2 units. I got the train home at 4pm. My eyes are now terribly sore amongst all my other problems. Tuesday, Wednesday, Thursday and Friday my radiotherapy continued to be done but on the Wednesday my condition began to go downhill very quickly. I felt weak and could not eat or drink anything. I have many many problems and I fear for my immediate future. By the end of Wednesday evening, I could feel dehydration kicking in. I could not take any water, food or medication. Something had to go very wrong soon. I still attended my Radiotherapy sessions but inside the same radiotherapy was destroying me and nobody was helping me. On the Friday while I was having the treatment at 1.10pm in Electra 5, the staff noticed my condition and I asked for help. Things moved fast and I was admitted as a patient. I was in a bad state with many problems with potential life threatening issues. After all, I had not been eating, drinking or taking any meds in three days. Is it any wonder I was so sick now?

——— # # # ———

MONDAY MARCH 21st my radiotherapy was done as normal in Electra 5 at 9.45am. I am still a patient in Guys but I am in a ward of complete and utter f*****g arsesholes and w*****s, however I suppose beggars can't be choosers, especially in my position. For the rest of the week my treatment progressed but I still feel terrible and yes, I still want to die. This is certainly no type of life to live. Right now I have nothing good going for me. I now have an infection in my right arm after a dirty needle. Today, Monday 21st, I had an x ray of my swallowing. The radiotherapy has burned my throat inside and this moving x ray shows that my epiglottis is badly burned and damaged. I would love to stop this treatment now but what's the point as it's near finished. My chest hurts and it's full of phlegm etc.

——— # # # ———

TUESDAY MARCH 29th. A decision was taken to get some food into me. At my bedside, the dietician and a nurse inserted a feeding tube into my stomach via my nose and down my throat. No numbing whatsoever and it was pure hell getting it in its correct place. An x ray was used for its insertion in case it entered my lungs. It was however in the correct place and now food could be put into me at last. I look hideous with a yellow tube coming out of my stomach and up my throat and out of my right nostril. It is then outside and attached to the side of my face with a plaster. What must people think when looking at me. Cancer is now getting more revenge on me. I am now in the closing stages of this Radiotherapy and I can't say it's been fun.

——— # # # ———

SATURDAY APRIL 2nd 2016. WOHOOOOO. Today is Day 30 of my Radiotherapy. Thirty days that began promising me so much and look at what it gave me. I am now in a hospital bed being very sick, dehydrated and a yellow tube hanging out my nostril with its sole purpose being just to get liquid food into me. I hate myself and I hate life. I am begging to die in my sleep to rid me of pain but my lovely Gaz is my one reason now for living.

——— # # # ———

TUESDAY APRIL 5th 2016. I was discharged from Guys. I now have a machine at my bedside at home which I plug in at night and while I am asleep, it simply pumps 1500 calories into me. It keeps me alive but it is not fun at all. Also today the washing machine packed in. I now have district nurses popping in to check on me. I do not have a good history with district nurses. As far as I am concerned so many are crap and give a bad name to the good ones. I reckon that on the day the good Lord above was giving out life to human beings he made a few cock ups and to cover these errors he decided that the shit humans he created would be the ancestors of stupid asshole people known as district nurses. Okay, maybe they are good, but in my life I have only been sent the rubbish ones. Let me give you an example. Thursday April 7th 2016 I had a visit in afternoon from two district nurses. Gaz, my son, was with me and witnessed this. Two district nurses and one of them was in training. I think her name was Precious or Blessing or something like that but you get my idea of the scene. The trainee we will call Precious was making a few blunders and really didn't know what she was doing but as we survived the visit, I really was upset that she was breathing the same air as me and sharing the same space on planet earth as I was. As they were leaving by the front door with their car parked outside, Precious was the last to leave. After what happened next, the car became their getaway car. Precious said goodbye and the front door closed behind her. Then after a few seconds I heard a loud clatter inside the door as something hit the floor. Gaz and I went out and on the floor was my f*****g letterbox. Precious had pulled the door outwards by pulling the letterbox outwards and slamming the door shut. The letterbox had then fallen away as she pulled it so what did she do, yes you guessed correctly. She posted my f*****g letterbox back to me via the hole now left by the absent letterbox. She then probably ran to their getaway car to leave the scene of the crime. I never want so see her again as long as I live. There you go, that's why me and district nurses do not see eye to eye. If you want your house demolished, let me know as I have their contact number and they'll send Precious round to do a good wrecking job in record quick time. On Friday April 8th I had an appointment with Mr J which was cancelled by someone on his side again. Anyhow, I do not want to see this man ever again after what he done to me.

——— # # # ———

WEDNESDAY APRIL 13th 2016. I had an INR check in morning and in afternoon I had an appointment in Guys at 12 noon. This appointment is with the Dietetic Dept to see how I am after all the treatments. They soon saw the state that I was in which was awful. Most days are bad now as a result of this Radiotherapy. I think to myself now, was it all worth it to put my body through hell? I have peripheral neurapathy, tiredness, sore throat and therefore totally unable to swallow. The phlegm in my lungs etc is thick and difficult to get up. It's choking. As the month progressed, I got so, so sick.

——— # # # ———

On WEDNESDAY APRIL 20th 2016, I had an appointment to see Theresa my consultant at 3.40pm. She is aware that the only way getting food into me now is via the machine at night, into my feed tube via nostril into throat and stomach. My pain relief is with morphine but this is now changed to Oramorph. Theresa then told me that Oncology and in particular Mr J had f****d up big time and that a formal letter of apology was being prepared to be then sent out to me. She would review me in a couple of weeks. On April 22nd, I had an appointment to see Dr C to review my pain control. She too, was visibly shocked with the state of me. My Oramorph was increased and was my Soluble paracetamol was slightly increased as well. As the month drew to a close, I again saw Theresa on April 27th at 9.50am followed by Dr C checking my pain. Theresa only wanted to see how I was coping but she soon realised that things were not improving at all.

——— # # # ———

On MONDAY MAY 2nd. Gaz made me a cuppa tea. This was sore but was also the first taste of tea in many, many months. It was okay but not wonderful but I had to see what level, as regards swallowing, I was in right now. Tonight also Gaz and his girlfriend went on holiday for just under two weeks. On May 4th a nurse came to change dressings holding my nasal tube in place. No letterbox fiasco this time as the nurse was civilised and knew how to close a door properly.

——— # # # ———

FRIDAY MAY 6th today, feel a little better but not out of the woods yet. However my other problems are not going away and will not for some time to come. Monday May 9th. Today is a very bad day with all my pain and problems are back full. My body shocks are also getting more frequent as is the soreness in throat and peripheral problems. I want to die peacefully now.

——— # # # ———

WEDNESDAY MAY 11th. I had an appointment in Guys at 1.40pm to see my consultant. Theresa expects me to have the nasal gastro tube in for at least another six to eight weeks. Despite all my current problems, Theresa is reasonably happy with my progress, even if I can't see it. She wants to see me back in clinic on June 8th. Can you imagine what I am going to go through between now and then. My throat is now unbearable. What am I gonna do in the name of God? Life is hell. Please someone help me. I can't put up with this much longer. The thing is, nobody understands what I am going through unless they themselves are going through it or are helping someone through it. One more thing, before I pass by it and not mention it. The fakes, oh yes. the f*****g fakes. They are still all around me and not showing any sign of going. I am however, one step ahead of them, always have been and always will be. As we approach the end of the week it's Friday 13th and I have an appointment at 11.15am with speech and language in Harris Hospice building near Orpington Hospital. It is actually a place where the Oncology community head and neck team have regular clinics, so cancer patients with head and neck cancer that live locally do not have to go to Guys to be seen. Of course, I still have to go to Guys to see my consultant and have treatment. This place is, where I think I already told you some time back I had an appointment, did not read the small print. I assumed it was to put my name down for the hospice to spend my last days on this earth but it was in fact to attend one of these clinics. In a way I was relieved when I realised my real purpose for being there in the first place.

——— # # # ———

SATURDAY MORNING 14th ... Gaz and his girlfriend came back from holiday. I am so glad to have them back home beside me. I fear getting sick or worse when my nearest and dearest are not near me. I still cry however every single day at the way this cancer is destroying me. The treatment of course is also wiping me out. Every day I think about the end of my life and all that may happen to me towards the end. I have, as you know, already planned my funeral as I have been told that I will be heavily sedated at the end. My family know about my planned funeral and it's all in a white envelope. All they have to do is simply open the envelope and follow the instructions inside as to what I want done. This way makes it easier all round for everyone. I make one extra request though and that is that my Gaz is the only one that can alter anything. As regards my health problems, I do notice that the phlegm is easing off. My next scan will be crucial as the treatment will of course be based on any scan results. I must then again decide to accept any treatment offered or not. My quality of life is important and my consultant will also be basing her treatment decision on that as well. It's a shit choice and a cruel choice but it must happen. I can certainly not go through all the past treatments all over again. As the month of May draws to a close my life, as regards this cancer, seems to be less intensive nowadays. In the past year or so it is gone from daily incidents to weekly or so. Whatever happens, I will still put it all down in a diary and then into this book. My writing now will be on a month by month basis. Monday 23rd and I have a 2.35pm appointment in Orpington Hospital with Mr P or one of his team. Again, they tell me that they will do nothing because of my situation. In other words they will do nothing because if they do something like a new knee then if I die it will be a waste of their money and knee sockets. If they are that worried about spare parts, I will sign anything that allows them to have the parts back from the crematorium after my funeral. What a bunch of bastards to not do anything. On the 27th I attended a speech and language appointment in the clinic in Harris Hospice near Orpington Hospital. I am also now planning a return trip to Skiathos in Greece. Skiathos is without doubt in my mind one of the loveliest places on this earth. I have been going there since the 1980's and I just love the place and the people there. It was also where I met Milena. This time in June, I will be returning there with my partner. On the 31st I booked in online for Skiathos on Tuesday June 14th. I can't wait to go there as this may be a sign that my health is improving.

——— # # # ———

JUNE 2016 is here and on WEDNESDAY JUNE 8th 2016 I had an appointment in the PRUH for INR and in afternoon at 3pm with Speech and Language and at 4pm an appointment with Theresa my consultant. My speech and language appointment went okay as it was basically just to see me swallowing etc, which is not really happening as I have a tube into my nose and down to my stomach. We updated my medication which is now Oxycodone, Pregabalin, Carbocistine, Diflam spray, Hydrogen Peroxide, Domperidone anti-sickness, Bisoprolol, Vitamin B, multivitamins, Nicorandil, Paracetamol and Thiamine. What a list eh! My face is now very swollen as fluid drainage in face etc is not working properly. Theresa has referred me to the Lymphoedema team. Theresa has said that I should have a Pet Scan in about 12 weeks time to check on the cancer and my next appointment will be to get the results of that scan. The month of June progressed and things have not changed. I hate this cancer and what it's done to me. It's changed me and I hate people and I hate myself.

——— # # # ———

SATURDAY JUNE 11th was our Street Party in my road. I had help to organise it from some neighbours who also brought out their own home cooked food. It was a great day all round.

——— # # # ———

TUESDAY JUNE 14th. My partner and I flew to Skiathos. I got a doctor letter to bring all my medication on holiday in the plane with me. I had to judge the amount of pain relief and take enough to get me through. I took a chance and even though I took travel Insurance, I could not afford the cost of cover for my cancer. I also had to take my feeding machine, syringes, spare adapter feed tubes.

I also took packs of liquid food with me and pack it securely in suitcases as it was too big and had to go in the hold of the plane. When I reached the apartment at the Marina Hotel in Skiathos, I got such a shock. I did not count on the baggage handlers in Gatwick. Two bags of food had burst in one of the suitcases and had damaged and covered some of my holiday clothes. I tried washing them over the next two days but they were stinking and stuck together. The holiday however was great, apart from the fact that every day and night when my partner and I went out to restaurants, she ate normally and I had to just sit there, night after night, and just looked on with a tube hanging out of my nose. What a sight. I could not eat or drink and I felt totally alone and lost in my own world. I never did see anyone else in the same position like me during the entire holiday. It was hell just sitting there day after day and night after night but I was content as I never thought I would see Skiathos ever again. Maybe after the holiday, my thoughts and health may improve. I want to return to Skiathos again if I can, please God. On June 17th, my pain relief in Oromorph ran low and I had to see an emergency doctor to give me pain patches. It cost me 62 euros. This is where I miss the NHS. Because I did not have enough pain relief, I had to ration it and therefore my pain increased daily. My holiday was in danger of being ruined but I took enough Paracetamol to ensure that it was a good holiday. The Radiotherapy has certainly done a lot of damage to me. On 21st we returned from Skiathos. When I weighed myself I found out that I lost 5 kilos in 7 days in Skiathos and I was also glad to get my Oxycodone pain relief which I had here at home in the house. On 22nd I had more appointments in Guys. At 12 noon was an appointment with Becky in Speech and Language. She is happy with my progress. On 23rd I had an appointment with Lymphoedema clinic. My facial fluid moves from one side to the other. However when I am plugged into my food and machine at night, I am lying all night on my left side. In the morning the left side of my face is very swollen from fluid and it takes all day to balance the swelling out. In the clinic I was given a Hereford collar to wear to force the fluid out of my facial areas but of course it all returns and swells up by the end of the day. I have a scan in a couple of days, what news will it give me, I dread it all. On 25th I had a problem with my feeding tube, as it blocked up. On 26th my N G Feed tube was totally blocked and I had to go to A and E to have it replaced. I was discharged from the PRUH at 1.30am on 27th.

——— # # # ———

WEDNESDAY 29th. In St Thomas's for my all important Pet Scan at 11.30am. JULY 4th 2016 I drank a full cup of tea today, something which I have not done in a long long time. Wednesday July 6th 2016. Today I see Theresa at 5.10pm. I have requested hospital transport. What a fiasco. Transport was booked to collect me at 2pm to be on time for my scan results. However the transport came at 5pm and only got to Guys at 6.20pm. I phoned ahead to explain and they said all was okay. When I got there most of the team was gone but I eventually met someone. My news was very good, all the cancer is no longer visible in my neck and throat area so the Radiotherapy has worked. It does not say that it is gone, only says that it is no longer visible. There is a 2mm spot in my right lung however. July 9th, Gaz and his girlfriend are decorating their new home. My days are now getting better. I still have many problems but my energy is coming back slowly, a good sign of things to come.

——— # # # ———

ON WEDNESDAY JULY 20TH. I had an appointment to see Theresa in Guys at 3pm. Theresa's clinic always runs late so it was about 3.40pm before I was called in. Beforehand I had my height and weight taken. The waiting room, as usual, is packed solid, all races and creeds but all with cancer. Today is a good day overall and my energy levels are definitely returning. I say returning but it will be a long time before fully normal but of course any future treatment will stop all that and we will then be at square one again. I can't win, can I? Theresa however is pleased with my response, as the head and neck area is now looking better. She is considering requesting a flouroscopy test which is basically a moving x ray of my swallowing and any problems with it. The month of July progressed. On 22nd I saw speech and language in Harris Hospice clinic in Orpington. Phlegm is easing but I am still nervous to drink via the mouth any tea or water. If you remember, I think I told you that my Epiglottis is damaged by the Radiotherapy and the danger is liquid can go down the wrong way and if that happens I can get a chest infection. Chest infections with a low or non existing immune system can sometimes result in death. Overall, taking into account Theresa's clinic and Speech and Language, it looks like there is currently nothing nasty showing up in my head and neck area, there is however, a slight raised area of concern in my right lung. I am still concerned slightly but a Pet Scan is the only way to sort this all out. On Sunday 24th I tried Minestrone soup. It was hell and so spicy and blew my head off. It will not be normal for many months if not years to come.

——— # # # ———

TUESDAY JULY 26th 2016, tried porridge. It tasted foul. I also have a new problem which is balance problems. I never know what to expect next. The fluid in face and chin is very bad and showing no sign at all of easing off. I remember being told in the early stages that this fluid retention problem could take years to recover itself. I am totally dependent on my liquid feed into me via tube and machine. This is no way to live, no way at all. When am I going to get better and cease to be in this awful existing life?

——— # # # ———

The month of AUGUST 2016 began just like last month. Body shocks, Peripheral problems, Balance problems, Sore throat, Feeding tube and now a new problem of dropping things.

——— # # # ———

TUESDAY AUGUST 6th my feed tube is giving problems and on the 7th I went to A and E dept at 3.45 in afternoon. Tube was replaced and I was sent home again at 6.30pm. I was advised to put lemonade through the tube to keep it from blocking up. The blocking up was caused by stomach acids attacking it as to the stomach the tube is an alien and should not be there. This will always be the case. Of course we are now in the month of AUGUST and the weather is good and hot.

——— # # # ———

THURSDAY AUGUST 11th 2016. I had spare cash of £30 in kitchen. It's been there for many months as emergency cash for anything. This evening I discovered that it is now missing and immediately I think I know who took it. The thief is a female and not family, dirty thieving bitch. I have decided to leave £10 on the mantle piece over the fire as a trap. Let's see how long it lasts as I will be checking every day even every hour. She is a low down dirty thieving bitch and I will prove that she took it. OKAY. Let us carry on and not get too upset, however as soon as that £10 walks from over the fireplace, then the shit will hit the fan big time. I certainly do not need a thief near me. My health certainly has not improved. I still have the same problems and now I am dropping more things than before. The pain is difficult to control but it is getting there in being controlled. The phlegm is easing off. How much longer will this hell last for me? Will it be death or will it be a lifetime of treatment and an uncertain quality of life? Every morning now I wake up and I have no idea how good or how bad the day will be ahead for me. What I have noticed are the body shocks. My body jolts like an electric shock is put through me. It's like when I was a kid back in Ireland all those years ago and coming home from my primary school in the afternoons and me and my school mates as a dare would touch the electric fences used by farmers on the ditches to stop the cows in the fields escaping. It was guaranteed that this would happen at least once a week. I can promise you this, I never developed an immunity from these electric fences so the weekly torture was always guaranteed in all weathers and I spent many years in that Kilcoleman National School. God, all those innocent days as a child growing up in the country, little did I know then that I would be dying from f*****g stupid shitty bastard cancer. I was an innocent child leading an innocent life then. I dare say that there are thousands like me in the same situation. I'm diverting a little bit now but one more thing that I will never forget is that I have always been a religious man and my faith is important to me but back in Ireland also as a kid, I liked going to mass and there were masses on Saturday evening at 6pm and then on Sunday at 10am and 6pm. However there was one thing and I might go to hell for this. It's funny but true. All the masses were, near enough, lasting just under the hour long but me and many catholics like me were attracted to the idea of the priest who perfected the 20 to 25 minute mass. No strings attached, no sermon or speech rammed down our throats. Guess what too, if there was ever a sermon at mass, then Monday morning a teacher was guaranteed to ask you what was the sermon about. The best way to avoid it was to get the mass without the strings attached. That was my excuse but God Bless my parents, they sometimes got the longish mass and then I had to take in the sermon or face the shitty consequences at school on Monday morning if I failed the sermon question. Sick on Mondays sometimes worked but it was a risky habit to adopt in West Cork and the catholic fuelled slaps on a Monday morning. Master O Farrell was my teacher and he gave me and many others a lift to school in the mornings. Later in the morning the same guy would slap the shit out of me if the sermon slipped my mind. Right that's enough of that, let's get back to this cancer problem that I have. August 22nd 2016 and as we approach the end of this month the weather is warm and I have enough energy now to paint Gaz's bedroom duck egg blue. This is a good sign but I am still not forgetting that I have terminal cancer and it's only to control it a little as it is not curable in any shape or form whatsoever. Becky my speech and language has told me that my feed tube is more than likely long term. I have every intention that I will not have it for life. I am a fighter but sometimes it does get to me. Today is August 23rd and I have a new problem in that my eye is swollen badly and as a result I missed a podiatrist appointment in Orpington. My right eye is practically totally closed where the fluid in my face moved up into my eye while asleep. It will take all day for it to move down. They will reschedule my appointment. My face looks swollen and awful. My balance problems are also pretty bad as are the swollen feet. Friday 26th is today and a 1.30pm appointment with Yvonne my Dietician in Harris Hospice clinic. All is okay as it was just a progress check. I got home and paid £1,031.00 for 45 Christmas panto tickets. Weather is still hot today and my partner is admitted to A and E in Woolwich. It is okay, it seems to be a kidney infection. Today also my left eye socket is swollen where the fluid has gone in a new direction. I still look hideous and people will look at me strangely like they did last week with my other eye. I can still see the £10 note near football trophy over fire. Obviously I will only check of it still there when this certain person is in the house and that person is here today. At 10.50 this morning Dr Parker saw me in his doctor surgery and referred me to a physio Wednesday 31st I have an appointment in Guys at 10.30am. I saw Becky my dietician and she is discussing with me the possibility of moving the feed tube from where it is now into nostril and moving it to my abdomen and directly into stomach. It's called a PEG or a RIG. Today also I received a letter from PALS which is an apology from Mr J and Oncology for not looking after me properly and missing important scan etc. I am not happy with this letter of explanation but what can I do, I need these people. They are all very good but someone f****d up somewhere. I think it is best if Mr J stays out of my way from now on and we leave it at that. There are so many great people looking after me, my CNS's Claire and Hannah. Then there is my consultant Theresa, I love them all so much. At the meeting with my dietician, I asked if a surgeon could operate and repair. Straight away my partner erupted and said "forget it, nobody can help you so it is best if you forget the whole idea". Everyone in the room including me is shocked by my partner's outburst. It suddenly seems to me that she may not want me to get better. Maybe I am imagining it but I am surprised she said this and I can't help thinking what I think she means or wants to happen to me. I hope I am wrong thinking this as I want to live for a long time yet. Why did she say it? Did she say it just to make me aware that any attempt to operate would probably not work anyway. Let's see eh!

——— # # # ———

Good morning all. IT'S THURSDAY SEPTEMBER 1st 2016 and I am having one of those wonderfully clever PET Scans' in St Thomas's Hospital at 10.30am. My partner was with me at Guys for support. At least she can't do any objections in this scan. She is in the waiting room while I'm being scanned for a couple of hours. We got home from the hospital and I then had to take her home. I popped in next door to speak to the builder in Number 36 to ask him to move his van. I took her home and on my return here home later that evening, I discovered the £10 note had gone. There was only one person in that room while I was next door. I phoned her at home and simply asked if she had moved any money as it has gone. Her reply was that she had moved no tenner. Instant self conviction as I never mentioned to her the note denomination. I told her to go to hell. A few days later with a friend of mine, I took some clothes she had here over to her sister. Her sister then told me that she knew that she took from me and that she, my partner who had been a big part of my life, was the one who did me harm and now I know why small amounts of money disappeared. The biggest shock was that I now know that there was a big plan to be a close part of my life and not for me to get better but me to get very, very ill and she get a lot of my money etc. So she didn't want me to get better and now I know why, in the room that day, she objected to me getting better when the plan all along was for probably for me not to get better and guess who wanted to benefit from my decline in health. What a bitch. Karma will bite back. Guaranteed. Let me tell you that there are bad, bad women out there. Now, how is that for a revelation in this book. See all and tell all! It had to be told as it is all part of my life, my health, my cancer and anything that is associated with it.

——— # # # ———

MOVING ON NOW! MONDAY SEPTEMBER 5th 2016. The year is flying by and surely you, as a reader, must notice that compared to last year and the previous year, there is far less happening as regards daily serious events with my cancer. I hate those fake people still and it's especially annoying when they continue to be fake but have no idea that I know what they're doing. I say to myself now and again that surely they can't be all that stupid, but yes they are that stupid. Let them carry on then I have no tales to tell you today about school and church when I was a kid. I recollect more and more now the number of people that I know from work who have retired because of ill health and it is normally down to heart attacks and stress associated with the job as a bus driver. Cancer is so f*****g devastating when told but we've been through all that. I do however think about my predicament every day and what will happen to those I leave behind. In a way for me it's okay because when I die, that's it. Those that I will leave behind, well that's when their nightmare actually continues. Their nightmare began the day that I was diagnosed and it will in effect never end. They support me in every way and help me from diagnosis day and the moment that I die is when it actually gets worse for them. I worry every single day about my Garreth and he worries about me. I really hope that his pain will not be too much when I do pass away.

——— # # # ———

Okay, where are we, oh yes, Wednesday SEPTEMBER 7th 2016 and today I am seeing Theresa my lovely consultant. It is now four and a half months since the end of radiotherapy to the head and neck area, and the uptake in cancer cells is reduced. However, the lung tumour is now 8mm in size. No more treatment for now but it will be monitored. Theresa has also agreed to putting a RIG tube into the belly area and directly into the stomach. No more tube in my face, no more stares from people while out shopping etc. No more ignorant parents pulling their kids aside when near me and loud whispers of "that man is sick, he should be put away in hospital and away from the public" or what I once heard when a child looked at me in Tesco in Orpington and said to an older person with them "Is that man sick". The older person replied "yes and he's dying". It is horrible hearing things like that being said. They're correct though. I am sick and I am dying but maybe not too soon hopefully. Gaz was with me and he too was very happy with what I heard from Theresa. We left the room and made our way to the train and eventually home. Swelling very clear to see its big in face, under chin and right eye socket. Sometimes it's the left socket but never both at the same time. Right now I could make a living scaring the wits out of people. Thursday 8th, I saw podiatrist and I was discharged from their system. My toes are well and all is healed okay. At home I am keeping busy by collecting signatures from residents of my road to improve the parking in the road. I like all this and it keeps me busy. My friends John and Cheryl are true friends and help me a lot. John is going to pop around some time to tidy up the bushes in the garden etc. The letter I got from Oncololgy and Mr J apologising to me and promising to improve things has already proved that it is useless and means nothing. Today, Thursday September 15th, they sent me an appointment for December 7th for a PET Scan in St Thomas's and also at the same time to see Theresa in Guys to get the same scan results. How can that make sense? They will have to change one of them. Friday 16th. I got a phone call from Theresa's secretary to keep the scan date on December 7th and an appointment has been made to see Theresa on the 14th. Glad it is finally sorted.

——— # # # ———

SATURDAY SEPTEMBER 17th. On a personal matter, no contact from the alleged thief . As for my illness, my face is now very hideously swollen. My energy levels are now good. John and Cheryl came on Sunday 18th and cut my garden. My good mate Lizzie popped over on Monday 19th to see me. On Tuesday 20th, I attended Orpington Hospital at 10.15am to have a knee brace fitted. I'm surprised that they are actually spending the cost of that on me. Thursday 22nd I was in Guys to see Mr J. I do not like this guy but he wants to see me. He is ruthless and does things that are not popular. He disagreed about my liquid food and said I was depending on a bag of chemicals to live. He then acted out of order and pulled out the feed tube which was still in nostril. I was so shocked about he being ruthless in this action. He did this against the advice of my consultant and just proves that he does not give a shit and loves the glory etc. I hope he hasn't made another blunder but I think he has done something wrong again. Because I am not taking anything in via the tube, I now fear that I will have some weight loss. I got home fearing for my future. Friday 23rd I saw Sam the physio in Harris Hospice clinic. I also met Rebecca from Speech and Language all to see how I was coping without the N G Tube. Saturday 25th I knew it would happen. I'm not taking in much food and water intake is difficult as ever because my throat is sore. I feel that I am getting weaker as a result and I will be very sick in a couple of days. Then it happened, I collapsed on the floor and the last that I remember was that it was 5pm. I thought I would have at least lasted a couple of days, instead it was a matter of hours. I woke up at 7pm. I realised that I was getting seriously ill and knew that I had to pack a bag quickly and get myself into hospital as soon as possible. I dialled 999 and was told that it was a 50 minute wait. I texted a neighbour. She looked after me until the ambulance crew arrived. I was taken to the PRUH A and E. I was in cubicle 8 and was told that I was dehydrated and had a chest infection. The chest infection was with me because without the tube something I swallowed and gone down the wrong way and I aspirated. All because of Mr J and his latest blunder. He has now prolonged my suffering even more. I now really detest this guy, this lone ranger, this ruthless so called consultant. Theresa will be really upset with this latest incident. In the PRUH they put me on fluids via drip and of course more pain when they put the tube back into me via nostril again, yes the N G Tube is back in. An x ray confirmed that it was in the correct place. I was on a trolley in A and E until late next day evening which was a Monday. They moved me on Monday evening and as I was being moved to AEU it was shocking to see that there were 6 ambulance crews with their patients on trolleys. That is disgraceful, six crews off the road and waiting for their patients to be seen to. I would not forget this day in a hurry. It was Monday September 26th 2016 and I was in the Princess Royal University Hospital. Then I remember a pensioner getting a urine bottle from a nurse and all he said was, "what's this for, did they forget to build the f*****g toilets?" I had to laugh at what he said. In AEU I certainly had a rough experience. No pain killers given to me because of lack of staff. Next to me was a guy called Ricky on detox. Opposite me was a lovely poor guy called Francis who was confined to bed. Then there was Peter who was a retired Saville Row tailor. He had some great stories to tell me and to anyone who listened to him which I did as the other listening choice was the guy on detox. However, the Saville Row tailor was posh and did look down on everyone in the ward and on his visitors. That night the proverbial happened to Peter as he shit and pissed himself. Not so posh now Mr Peter are you? No you are not. His wife was posh too and had a foreign accent. I would love to have told her that Peter shit himself, but I didn't. I remember when it happened, Peter said to the nurse he didn't get to the bed pan and piss bottle in time. I laughed my ass off when the nurse told him that there was no pan or bottle nearby. Peter said nothing. Thursday night 29th nearly discharged but did not in the end. On Friday 30th however I was discharged in the evening. I felt sorry for Ricky and took his clothes home and washed and ironed them. I brought them back next afternoon. I wanted to do for someone what they might do to me. My great neighbour Paul took me home again after dropping Ricky his clothes off. I then noticed that the hospital staff had nicked my pill crusher and swapped it for a white hospital one. Thieving bastards. On Saturday October 1st at 9.48am was my appointment with my GP to have a flu jab. I am tired and recovering but tonight is a family reunion in Barnham. My Aunt Leonore is having her birthday party and I am going to it whether I am sick or not. She is 90 years old and such a lovely lady so it's a big event in her life. My problems are many but my Oxynorm pain relief is a great help.

——— # # # ———

MONDAY OCTOBER 3rd 2016. I attended the warfarin clinic for the last time at 10am. No more trips to this clinic. My INR is 1.2 and from now on my blood thinning is every day self injecting into my belly with Clexane pre filled syringes. I know what's ahead. My belly will me full of bruises on both sides as I will have to do alternate sides by pinching the skin to not feel the needle going in and then let go as I pull the needle back out after its contents are gone into me to thin my blood out and thus prevent my blood clotting. Guys have delivered to me a machine to reduce the build up of phlegm in my chest etc. I forget the name of it but it is good. OKAY. I just remembered. it's a Nebulizer. Noisy but good. Just to update you now, my current problems are as follows: Body shocks, facial swelling with lots of fluid called Lymphedema, tiredness, numbness and tingling in feet, toes, and fingers. I have major balance problems, My NG tube which was recently put back in via my nostril, Phlegm in chest etc, sore throat and problems swallowing. On Thursday 6th 2016, I had an appointment in Guys with Counselling. I had enough of these pricks in the past and in particular M. S. That woman drove me absolute bloody crackers and a repeat was not for me. I have enough problems. On Friday October 7th 2016 was my 59th birthday and I was to see Sam the physio in the clinic at Harris Hospice at 11.15am. I was also due to see at same meeting Becky of Speech and Language and Yvonne my dietican. I have no problems with these people, in fact I think a lot of them.

On October 10th, Oncology confirmed that my Feed tube surgery to have it put into my stomach via abdomen would happen on the 20th in the PRUH. The liquid food however stinks and makes such a mess everywhere. The clexane has as yet not caused much bruising but soon however it will happen. To keep myself busy I organised a survey in the road to see how many residents objected to the current parking problems. The result was expected to be high in favour of council restrictions on outside people parking in our road. The results would be in a matter of days. Saturday 15th and Liam, my brother, has messaged me to say he is coming to see me this coming Monday evening. I'm looking forward so much to this as he is having problems coming to terms with the idea that I am going to die from this cancer. A friend of mine who would later be a gold digger and a fake messaged me to say she was in hospital after taking pills. I have enough problems but I visited her, even though I guessed at the time that she was a fake but had not confirmed. I was one step ahead of her but she didn't know this. She has many problems but I am not judging her yet. Monday 17th October, my fridge packed in, bloody hell, that's all I need. Gaz found one in Currys and sent me the link which allowed me to order it and have it delivered on Wednesday. Liam arrived and he looks well compared to the last time. Liam and I stayed up chatting till 2.30am. We had a great catch up and I think now he does realise that my cancer is as bad as it is and a cure is not happening. Tuesday 18th. Liam had an early shower and I was up at 9.30am to get milk from my spare fridge in my garage at the rear of my garden. We had another great chat and now I realise what a crazy busy life he has in his job. He has a lot of danger in some countries that he works in. He left at 1pm to catch a flight back to Amsterdam. I miss him now that he has left. We hugged each other something that we haven't done in many years.

——— # # # ———

Wednesday 19th my fridge arrived. Happy days.

——— # # # ———

Thursday 20th OCTOBER 2016. Today is NG tube removal day and new one into my belly. No clexane blood thinning last night and for a couple of days afterwards in case of bleeding. I went to look for someone to give me a lift into the PRUH for my procedure which is called a "RIG", but of course those that promised me in the past that they would be there for me were nowhere to be seen so I had no alter native but to add them to my growing fakes list. A local neighbour Neelima took me into the hospital and even though she was busy, she took 15 minutes off what she was doing and took me into the hospital. Thank you Neelima. xx. The procedure was abandoned because my heart rate dropped and I was put in Farnborough Ward overnight for observation. Friday 21st, I was discharged in late afternoon with same tube in my nose still and not very happy with the whole thing at all. They will try another time soon I hope. My neck muscles are now a cause for concern. They are weak and my head is tilting forward a lot now. The parking on the road issue is in (YES: 57), (NO: 30) and (ABSTAIN: 22). Now I have to give these to the council as requested by them.

——— # # # ———

SATURDAY 22nd a friend, who now appears to be a fake, was discharged from hospital and visited me in the evening with a stupid small dog. That is one ugly vicious temper wa***r of an excuse for anything associated with the canine world. I have seen rats bigger than this little piece of shit. She left later with that ugly dog. The weather is cold today too. Sunday 23rd I went up to see Gaz and his girlfriend in their new place. I had tea, water and ate a half a stuffed pepper. Thanks Gaz for cooking and letting me try normal food again. I think it may be a turning point in my eating normally eventually. The clexane injections now are causing bruising to develop in my belly on both sides. It looks like I've been kicked in the belly. I do also find it difficult to sleep at night.

——— # # # ———

On TUESDAY 25th I had no alternative but to report the theft of money from me by my ex partner to her manager, because she looks after vulnerable people. She is allegedly the one who steal from me and I had to do it. Her manager would investigate immediately and as far as I am concerned I'm glad I have done it because there may be other victims. I am a cancer sufferer and look what happened to me by her hands who is potentially, slowly dying. Her family may also hate me but I was not the thief, she is allegedly the thief and the evidence is overwhelmingly obvious. Today also the weather is a little milder. As we approach the end of the month of October, My facial swelling is now very noticeable. I tried to eat porridge but it failed but I do notice that my energy levels are getting gradually better now. Weather is cold now a bit more today. Saturday 29th, energy levels have crashed today. Clocks go back by 1 hour tonight.

——— # # # ———

MONDAY OCTOBER 31st. Trick or treat tonight. This is one of those events where all the kids on the road go around with their parents. I did not expect to be alive to witness this event. There are so many events during the year now that I should not be alive to see, and it's very strange now that they are happening and I am still here. Trick or treat, bring it on and I love witnessing it and please God I will be here again next year 2017. My voice is now distorted a little and my neck is now really bent forward even more now.

——— # # # ———

TUESDAY NOVEMBER 1st 2016 and I am slowly introducing solid food, but as soft as possible of the date to do the procedure to put the RIG in to me. Wednesday 2nd is very cold today. I feel good and washed all my white shirts in whitener to make them even brighter looking. I have a lot of feet numbness today which is dangerous when driving.

——— # # # ———

SATURDAY NOVEMBER 5th. I had nasty text messages from the alleged thief to which I never replied or reacted in any way. My eating of soft food is going well. All my listed problems continue to annoy me. I also heard today that Danny Baker the DJ is going into the Jungle in Celebrity etc. He also revealed that he is 6 years clear of Head and Neck Cancer which is the type of Cancer that I have, it makes it easier for me to take in, as he is 6 years clear and maybe I can get a little bit of remission too. My face is very, very swollen today. I have been told that this swelling from fluid could be for a long, long time, possibly years. Again, more nasty messages from the thief. I still did not react and will not in any way whatsoever. What a nasty person she is. Tuesday, November 5th and the boss of the thief phoned me to confirm that she is under investigation Now I know why she sent me those messages. Her boss advised me to go to the police, but I have already decided that it ends now.

——— # # # ———

WEDNESDAY NOVEMBER 5th 2016 and Trump is elected president in USA. My problems continue just like those in the USA. My phlegm is easing now and the Nebulizer Machine goes back on the 14th of November.

——— # # # ———

THURSDAY 10th at 1.30pm I saw Starr in PRUH about my Gastric Band. All is well and I am 74.1 kilos. I am back to see her on May 11th 2017, also found out that Ann, the voluntary helper in the clinic, had passed away. Lovely lady she was and always asked about me when I had appointments. My neck still bent forward but tomorrow, Friday 11th at 11.15am, I see Sam the physio in clinic at Harris Hospice. I also am seeing Rebecca and Yvonne. I need Yvonne to chase up the RIG procedure date.

——— # # # ———

MONDAY NOVEMBER 14th. I had my new blinds fitted in my conservatory today and in the afternoon I had a call from Guys to tell me that the RIG or PEG procedure will happen, possibly on November 24th. It will be done in Guys but I have to wait for a confirmation letter in the post. Today, the 15th, I had a Fray bentos pie, a tea and 2 pork pies to eat. Of course that was not in one sitting. It was over the course of the whole day. The usual problems continue and the weather is now cold.

——— # # # ———

FRIDAY NOVEMBER 18th was of course BBC Children in need. Then problems. At 10.30am my NG tube in my face got blocked. Only 6 days before I get a new type of tube in belly and this one gets blocked. I did my shopping and chemist etc and then went to A and E dept in the PRUH. During the procedure at the hospital, they messed up a little and put it into my right lung. After removing it and fitting it properly, I got home at 9pm that night. I never expected the tube to get blocked up so soon. It has only been maybe 4 weeks or s. On getting home I rested. It's been a long day. I again ask myself, when is it going to end. Monday 21st, I attended Orpington Hospital about my knee appointment. Now, if you remember the last time, they told me that they wouldn't do anything to my knee while there is a possibility that I would die and if that's the case then any work to repair my knee would be a complete waste of their time and any parts they might put into me, well guess what, they repeated their plan. Nothing to be done and could I come back in 6 months time, where they will review my situation. When I think about it, it's a win, win situation for them. If I die, then of course I do not come back and if I do come back, well they're going to send me away again anyway. It's a joke and I can't see myself wining this argument. My phlegm is now completely cleared up but my other problems continue. My eating and drinking is now much improved.

——— # # # ———

WEDNESDAY NOVEMBER 23rd. I have to go to Guys Hospital today to Blundell Ward before 5pm for my procedure tomorrow to fit my RIG feed tube in belly. Hospital transport picked me up at 1.30pm. The Nebuliser machine which was due back on the 14th December was now going back today. When transport picked me up and took me up to Guys, I was admitted to Esther Ward after I dropped off the Nebuliser Machine to the chest clinic. In Esther ward, I ended up in Bed 19 and surgery is planned for the morning. Tonight I was nil by mouth prior to the procedure. Also no clexane blood thinning tonight.

——— # # # ———

THURSDAY 24th I was prepared for surgery. For this procedure I was given a local anaesthetic only as it was required that I be awake for the whole procedure. I had to wear a gown and surgery began at 9.30am with a hole being made in my abdomen. All I could feel was pulling and tugging as the muscle in the stomach wall was breached with a small blade. The stomach is pulled towards my abdomen inside and is stitched or clipped to the inside of my abdomen wall. Then, and only then, is the tube pushed in through a track from outside and into my stomach. Inside it is then inflated with 3 mls of water to secure it in place, and is then secured on the outside to the abdomen with a small rubber securement ring. The work was finished and I was in recovery by 11.30am. Eventually I was back in bed 19. Gradually water is inserted through the new tube. It feels so different not having a tube in my face now. The pain in my belly was bad now. They decided that I should recover more so they are keeping me in here for another night. Hopefully home tomorrow now. Friday 25th, I was due to attend at Harris Hospice clinic to see Rebecca and Yvonne my Dietican. As well as Sam the physio, all at 10.30am and Sam at 11.15am. The RIG area is now very, very sore tonight. The dietican showed me how to clean and dress the wound. I was discharged at 5pm into the care of Patient transport who took me home. I was told to expect a car, but instead I got a patient transport ambulance doing several drop offs. It was cold and bumpy which was hurting me and my stomach wound. I can't forget that tonight I have a hole in my abdomen and stomach wall which was not there last night. I got home at 10pm and straight to bed. Tuesday 29th, I cancelled the appointment to the Lymphoedema clinic for 1pm and explained why. I can honestly say that this clinic really couldn't care less if I turned up here or not. Wednesday 30th the external stitches fell out. I phoned them and was told not to worry as it varies from patient to patient. It's still very sore, hope it gets better.

——— # # # ———

Well good morning all. It's DECEMBER and we are fast approaching the end of 2016. The month of December like the other months had varied incidents and problems associated with my cancer. The biggest shock of all is that I am still alive and fighting despite the consultants telling me that I should be dead. I must be doing something right. I will be very happy if I manage to finish my book before I pass away. My problems are still unchanged apart from the phlegm which is now all gone, food intake has increased, as is drinking normally. Bromley council are now collecting my Sharps bin as I need them.

——— # # # ———

MONDAY DECEMBER 5th 2016. Big shock this morning when I found out on Facebook that my ex partner had died suddenly. Enough said about that after all that has happened. Also this morning, I got all the paperwork together and went to the Civic Centre in Bromley and applied for my Blue Badge. For many months I have been turning it down as I thought other people needed it, well I've applied now for it as I need it now more than ever. My RIG site wound is leaking and being dressed every day now.

——— # # # ———

WEDNESDAY DECEMBER 7th 2016. Today I had a PET Scan in St Thomas's Hospital. Just in case anyone has forgotten what is involved in this scan, I am taken into a room and a canula is inserted. Then Radiation sugar is pumped in to the blood system and after a wait of 1.5 hours I am then taken to the scanning room and scanned. At first the head and neck area and then the rest of the body. I am then allowed to leave after the scanning team are happy with the images taken. Obviously no movement is allowed and nine times out of ten I get an itchy nose. Nothing I can do but to put up with it. I got hospital transport there and back. On Thursday December 8th I booked as usual, my 71 seats for Christmas Panto 2017, that's next year and I have every intention of being around for it. I also today changed the water in my RIG tube. Three mls is removed by syringe and is replaced immediately by another 3mls. This is the danger time as with no water in balloon, it is easy to pull tube out when nothing secures it in place. If the RIG tube falls out, The tube has to be pushed back in place via its track into the stomach. If that is not possible then I have 4 hours to get to A and E and get medical assistance to get it back in place otherwise the track closes up. If that happens then loads of problems appear and the situation then is bad and would need surgery all over again to get back to normal.

——— # # # ———

FRIDAY DECEMBER 9th 2016. It's Panto night in the Churchill Theatre in Bromley with Aladdin. Craig Reville Horwood was the baddie but was a good baddie, great acting and singing and loved by everyone at the show. I felt good before and after the show apart from the usual problems that I have. My problems will be with me for a long, long time to come. I met so many of my friends and workmates and their families. I have every intention of being at the Panto again next year. It's strange saying that because one year I'm gonna say that and the f*****g cancer will have taken me. Because all the Pantos that I get seats for are on a Friday night, the kids do not have to get up for school next morning. The same of course applies to the parents or carers etc. We all went home after a good night and I was totally satisfied that I can still do things like this that benefit my nearest and dearest. It gives me a purpose in life just like putting this book together, in this case entering daily things into a diary and then into this format. Okay as we approach the middle of December everyone of course is planning for Christmas and the New Year ahead. My eating is now good and is something that I could not imagine would happen this time last year. On Wednesday December 14th 2016, I attended Guy's Hospital New Cancer Centre. This is a brand new multi-million pound cancer centre. It's bright, clean and absolutely lovely. It is also a more relaxing place to be treated in. I got my appointment for 1pm but was seen about half an hour later than that. I was in Consultation Room 2 and was told that the 8mm tumour was now 10mm. There is also a new one that is 5mm in size. Adriana who is part of Theresa's team also told me however that this is classed as being stable and therefore no treatment is planned for me at this stage. This is good news but Adriana did say that it would eventually get worse. Gaz was with me at this meeting, as he always is, and of course like me is happy with my results. Gaz has gone through so much pain watching me since my diagnosis back in late 2013. That was a bad f*****g day for us both, but we've come a long way since then and Gaz has been with me every step of the way. Family is so important and I am lucky in that respect. Of course some members of my family still find it difficult to come to terms with the fact that I am slowly dying from my cancer. What a horrible shitty word is CANCER....

——— # # # ———

THURSDAY DECEMBER 15th 2016 and one dept in Guys that really has failed me is the Lymphoedema Department. Countless times they have called me to arrange either an appointment in their clinic or a phone call to me type of appointment. Most of the times they have failed to call me or they have cancelled the actual appointment at short notice. Today at 9am was a phone call appointment and sure enough nobody called me. I called them later in the morning and left a heated colourful message. It was not nasty or abusive but I did tell them what I thought of their treatment of me. Friday 16th, next day they called me to apologise for not phoning me. I again told them my opinion of them and their department. It was a one way conversation after that and I hung up. At 3pm they called me again to arrange another appointment for 2017 next year on January 3rd 2017. Today also I changed the water in the RIG balloon by myself. I was nervous of course by myself as when the water is not in the balloon, there is nothing keeping it in place. Anyhow I did it and all was well. Without making a list again, all my problems continued as before.

——— # # # ———

MONDAY DECEMBER 19th. Today is very cold and I done some shopping in Bromley, Christmas shopping. My new Blue Badge arrived in the post. It's strange getting this as this is actual visual confirmation that I am now disabled in the eyes of the law. Up to now I found it hard to take in that I am disabled. Being disabled is such a stigma to have attached to you. I have drawn the short straw in life and nothing will alter that. It is also strange to take in that I will die disabled. I also now believe that I have an infection in my RIG site. I attended my GP and a swab was taken of it. I will call him in a couple of days and pick up a prescription if required. As the month draws to a close the outside world of course is planning and preparing for Christmas.

——— # # # ———

WEDNESDAY DECEMBER 21st 2016, at 4.30pm had an appointment with the nurse in my GP Surgery who dressed the site. No results back yet so no sign of any antibiotics. Nutricia Homeward also today delivered less than usual as I am now eating near normal. I am trying to get in the calories and at the moment am probably getting in about 900 to 1100 calories per day now. On 22nd swab results revealed an infection in RIG which I already knew about. The Doctor gave me antibiotics to clear it up. Job done. My body now too feels the cold and now something completely new is cramp in both legs. I can feel it coming on which is a good thing as I need warning when driving. Today was my first bad one and I could feel it coming on about 15 minutes ahead of when it actually happened. I also did my last minute delivery of cards and presents in my road.

——— # # # ———

Well here it is DECEMBER 24th, Christmas eve, and I drove to Farnham to spend Christmas with Gaz, his girlfriend and her family. Christmas day was sad news that George Michael died, what a loss to music in general. Also on Christmas Day I was able to eat small amounts of everything, Of course, I forgot to tell you that Oramorph pain killer really helps. I have been using it for many many months now and it really helps. Of course I have to be careful not to drive when I take any Morphine and also now when going to Farnham. I really did have a lovely Christmas as Gaz was with me all the time.

——— # # # ———

THURSDAY DECEMBER 29th. I spent the day with Gaz as he had booked time off. I went on the train with him to London and back. I love his place and spending time with him. On Friday 30th, Oncology called me and an appointment for March 14th 2017 has now been changed to March 22nd 2017 at 2pm. Gaz is staying here with me tonight. My feet cramps are bad. Overall I had a great Christmas with the people that mean the most to me. Therefore on New Year's Eve DECEMBER 31st, I was at home but this is the way I want it. Gaz was out with his then girlfriend and they were together to welcome in the New Year 2017. So HAPPY NEW YEAR 2017 to you all. I have no idea what the world has in store for me and I suppose my parents said the same thing on October 7th 1957, the day that I was born. Every New Year's Eve I say the same thing for the year ahead. Good Morning 2017. I spent last night saying goodbye to the old year and saying a big Hello to 2017, the New Year. During my reflective moments last night and this morning, I had all the time to myself to really dig deep into the back of my mind and try to put together anything that resembles a thought or a memory from the past 12 months. They came flooding back to me, so many of them and each and every one of them on a personal mission to mess me up. The memories of that treatment were bad enough to make my day-to-day living a combination of torment, crying and panic attacks. Basically a repeat of what I've been through for the past since late 2013, when first diagnosed. I often think to myself and this is the scary surreal part of it all. Here it is, On that date back in late 2013, I was told by a medical person much more clever than me, that I had lumps and that they were cancerous. Who am I to disregard what a person of medical knowledge knows and tells me. That day my life fell apart and I had a fatal disease that I only ever read about other people having and consequently they would die and that was it. Now, however, things were different and I, in his opinion, was the one going to die. Ever since then when gruesome treatment began I am at the mercy of chemotherapy, Radiotherapy and all that it done to my body. Now for the big question and this goes through my mind every single day. What if they got it wrong and actually made a mistake from Day One and all my suffering to date is all because of a medical blunder? This terrifies me so much. All my sores, sickness, bleeding, in fact everything that I have gone through up to now could be all one hell of a rollercoaster ride all because of a mistake. My family, friends and I put through this because of something that should not have happened in the first place. It's the stuff of nightmares but I'm stuck with it. Back to present day and I guess there's no point in doing anything now, as all treatment is ongoing and what has happened has happened. My life has fallen apart and I'm stuck with it. One thing that will not change however is this, I hate healthy people because it's not fair that I am so ill and dying like this. Now I can assure you this, what I went through is not the normal activity of a person trying to enjoy a normal New Year celebration. What I went through was hell, a day to day hell and unless you are fighting cancer, you have no idea what it is all about. January 1st 2017 is basically what lies ahead for me so let's see what 2017 has in store for me. People say things can only get better. I wonder, can they?

——— # # # ———

JANUARY 3rd 2017. I had an appointment at 1pm with the Lymphoedema clinic. The Lymphatic system in my body is basically the fluid draining out of my body to be expelled eventually in the normal way. Radiotherapy in all the damage that it done to me was concentrated on my face and neck area so a lot of the damage to the drainage system in my body was concentrated on my facial and neck area. Ever since my radiotherapy sessions ending then the fluid in my face and neck is not draining properly, if at all. The neck and throat has to be massaged on a regular basis several times a day to force the fluid out of the area of throat etc. The fluid soon returns to the area so it is a constant battle to keep the fluid away as often as possible. As a result also of this clinic meeting I was advised to wear a chin strap daily while I am not outside of my home. I'm not surprised, it looks silly and strange and resembles a tampon under my chin area and neck. It's meant to force the fluid out of the area, which it does, but it soon returns. I can assure you that it's not for anybody of the general public to see. Today is also my ex partner's funeral and because of the circumstances of our break up, therefore I did not attend. Just to show that the new year has no difference to my body problems, I am still putting up with the following on a daily basis, peripheral problems, body shocks, cramps in both feet, occasional nose bleeds, facial fluid, nausea and sometimes vomiting. Apart from Oxynorm a lot of my medication now is via the mouth. The weather is frosty. Another problem that I have but it's a common daily problem. I worry a lot about my Gaz but it's a Dad worry and that will not change even though he is 26 years old and 27 on March 1st. On January 19th Rosie my nutrician nurse paid me a visit to check on my feed tube in abdomen at 11am. All is well so far with that tube. On the 21st I looked for the first time at "motability" cars for me to change to. On the 24th I made an appointment with Volvo in Orpington to look further at "motability"cars. On 27th I met Yvonne my dietician in clinic in Orpington at 2.15pm and also for the first time discussed the possibility of the feeding tube may actually be in for life. On Sunday 29th I had further car viewing appointments with "motability" Renault and BMW. I think however that Volvo may be the one that I will end up with. I am really looking forward to a new car. It feels like an exciting part of my life may be about to happen to me. Not a lot more is happening right now and it feels like not a lot is happening. Just to explain this, on February 10th at 1.30pm I had an appointment with Kate the physio but to be honest she could do more for me. The next day is Saturday 11th and Gaz and his girlfriend took me out to the West End to see "Book of Mormon". This just also shows that my health is good enough for me to go out to see a show in the West End in London.

——— # # # ———

MONDAY FEBRUARY 13th 2017. Despite what I've just said about how my health has improved, many people say to me on a regular basis that now is the time to do your bucket list. Many people have in fact been telling me since shortly after I was diagnosed to do this list of things that I have always wanted to do. I have always wanted to visit New York, USA in general, Vietnam, India, a hot air balloon ride. Get behind the wheel of a formula 1 car, complete my flying lessons which I had begun before I was diagnosed and holiday in St Lucia or my lovely favourite Skiathos. Shortly after I started treatment back in 2014 my bucket list probably went out the window anyway because of insurance costs and being too bloody sick to do it anyway. Another thing is when I think about it, is doing a bucket list actually giving in and doing things before a person dies. I don't want to die, who does? So the longer I go without doing the list could in effect mean then I shall go on living. Can you imagine if this was actually true. If my other train of thought was that I was not actually cursed with cancer and they misdiagnosed me then I have nothing to worry about. CANCER! Is one horrible shitty disease and an even shittier word. So here we are in the middle of February 2017 and I now have to soon make a decision about when this book will actually come to an end. I have no idea when my condition will again deteriorate further of if is actually going down that path. For all I know, and God forbid if it does happen, my health may even take a turn for the worse tonight, tomorrow, next week, next month or next year. I have absolutely no idea but my doctors have told me that as time progresses then my chances are decreasing all the time but I will have reasonable time to start closing off this book. If I do run out of time, all I actually want is to finish the book. My family have said that if need be then they will get it edited and published. Many people hide their cancer but, as you can see, I do not and have been very, very open about my cancer and my journey. I held nothing back and believe me it has been a f*****g nightmare. I have tried to carry on my life as normal as possible. I now have taken over as "Snow Friends" co ordinator in my road. This means that in preparation of snow and ice, I have been supplied by Bromley council with snow scoops and bags with a mix of salt and grit. I also do "street friends" where I have been supplied purple bags to give out to residents to collect up leaves in purple bags and then I arrange collection of same. What I am trying to say and show, is that my life goes on for me. It has been rough and is still rough but it's my way of coping with it. Same reason applies to why I organise Street Parties in my road and do the same for organising the annual Christmas Panto night out. So while I have the time to write, then let's get on with it. My left eye is swollen as is my face. I have an abscess in my left gum. However at the same time, I am eating near enough normal. If I only knew the future then now would be a suitable time to begin the conclusion to this book but I have no intention about doing that right now, maybe its like gambling with the future. It is in fact not that at all. I still have a lot to write and get out into the open and while I have appointments in my diary then my story goes on.

——— # # # ———

WEDNESDAY MARCH 1st is Garreth's 27th birthday. On Sunday March 5th I went to Farnham to celebrate the birthday of Gaz and his girlfriend's sister. Great to live normally. I only wish that this cancer never hit me so I could live normally. Friday March 3rd Guys Dental discharged me back to my own dentist. At least it shows that some bit of normality is maybe returning back to my life. The weather is now mild and March 8th today is a busy day today. I have an important Pet Scan in St Thomas's Hospital at 11am. No need to explain how the Pet Scan is done. I have had so many of them now. That night I had my first lesson to learn how to play the Ukulele. It's something different I suppose. March 17th and Happy St Patrick's Day to you all. One ex-work colleague Gary Reeves died suddenly. So young, but I couldn't go to the funeral. As for me, I have a bad headache also today. No idea why.

——— # # # ———

WEDNESDAY MARCH 22nd 2017 at 2.30pm I have an appointment in Guys to see my consultant and get the results of my latest Pet Scan. I am very, very tired today with no energy whatsoever. My appointment today was supposed to be on 15th but it was changed to 22nd. The result of this appointment was that Theresa was very pleased with my condition and a new scan would be arranged for 4 months from now. I have now got low volume lung disease and palliative care continues as before. On Monday March 27th, I put my car a VW Passatt on Auto Trader for £800. On 29th I had my last Ukulele lesson which was a basic course anyway. On Thursday 30th March, I collected my new car A Volvo V40, black in colour. Life seems normal but I cannot forget that I have bloody cancer. On April 6th 2017, I had a 4.15pm appointment with that man Mr J in Guys.

Monday April 3rd was an eventful day. I arranged to sell my old car to a group of men from Romania. I had to have my wits about me. Let me explain. I had the car advertised on Auto Trader. Auto Trader was very reasonable but anybody can turn up promising the best but like in my case intending to rip me off. Three males appeared around 7pm on this evening of April 3rd. I was having a rough day and of course they realised that maybe I was a soft touch. I already had my new car blocking in my old car and I had all the paperwork on hand. I was alone and did not want 3 strangers going through my house especially while I was unwell. They asked for the keys and started the engine. Soon the one behind the wheel started to rev the engine and asked me to reduce from £800 to £600. I refused and they gave me back the keys and left. I watched them drive away and within 10 minutes they returned with a wad of notes rolled up and they said that £800 was okay and again asked for keys. I checked the money and it was only £600. It looked good rolled up but lucky I checked. These bastards trying to rip me off and tried to take advantage of a terminally ill person. They asked me if I was sick and I told them directly my situation. They showed concern but I can easily spot a fake now so f*** them. Anyhow, they then said sorry about the money and soon found the correct amount of £800. I noticed that one of them was younger than the others and I moved my car and after exchanging a receipt and proper paperwork. It was so strange watching my car being driven away. The time was just after 8.15pm. At 9pm my mobile phone rang and it was police who had nicked them for speeding near London's Blackwall Tunnel. Behind the wheel of my car was the younger one who was just 16 years old, no licence and no insurance. I told the police what happened to me and that they bought the car around 8pm. Police agreed that I done everything correctly but that was it. I never heard from them again but I now also miss my car. However, I also think I was lucky.

April 6th I had a 4.15pm appointment to see Mr J. What a waste of time. It was only to keep him in the picture about my condition and he told me he was pleased with my progress and condition. So f*****g what. That man in my mind has caused me so many problems and he continues to annoy me ever since the day he operated on me and told me I was cured and of course I am certainly not cured. On April 7th 2017 was the date of another appointment at 1.30pm to see Sam my physio and Cate, yes Cate with a C, my CNS from Oncology. Cate never appeared and as for Sam my physio who was there but I am not happy with my progress. It feels exactly like the Physiotherapist one who also appeared just for the sake of it and to be honest I can see the physio going the same way. Guaranteed she is going to piss me off maybe not today but it will happen. On the 11th I had a gastric band check appointment in the PRUH. My weight is confirmed to be 76 kilos. I can remember the day in 2009 pre surgery when it was over 146 kilos. On 12th April, Nutricia who supply my liquid feed called and collected excess amount of food packets. On the 19th I had another Ukulele lesson. I finished the earlier course of lessons and this was a quick check up lesson. It went well but still not decided to take on more lessons. On April 21st I went to my old workplace to catch up with ex work colleagues. It was nice to meet up those who were there. There are however so many new faces there now. It was a good day to catch up with them. I miss this place so much and so many nice mates in here.

On 25th April was a dental appointment at The Lindens in Orpington and was told to come back in 6 months. They are now my new dentists. I say new but I had them before prior to my cancer diagnosis. On 27th at 11.20am was an appointment with my doctor who ordered a blood test. On the next day was 28th and at 1.30pm was another appointment with Sam my Physio. Another waste of time this physio visit. I popped into the doctors and so quick was the blood test result back that showed my white blood cells were very low. May 5th, the Lymphodema clinic cancelled the appointment. These people seem to be giving me the run around. May 12th at 11.15am was an appointment in Harris Hospice, now St. Christophers, to see Cate my CNS. Cate is new but is looking promising and very helpful in her new position. She is in the same job as Hannah and Claire and I adore these CNS girls, so human and so helpful. Cate cancelled at last minute but came out to the house to see me.

Moving on now, it is Monday May 22nd 2017 and I had an appointment on Monday 22nd at 3.15pm to see about my knee. Again nothing will be done while the possibility of me dying might waste their time and metal bits in my knee. Basically this might seem funny but it's true, If I live, the threat of my dying stops any work and of course if I die the same applies. They still want to see me but I have no idea why? Now have you noticed one thing and this has happened before. My health is not great but things have levelled out. There are less incidents happening now again but as things happen there may be many days apart from one incident to the next so as you may have noticed that there are so so many pages for the early stages of my cancer journey being recorded and noted, whereas now there are far less pages for any incidents over the past 12 months or so. Already we are approaching the month of June 2017 but first let me tell you about the last day of May in 2017. On that day, the 31st May I had what I thought would be the most embarassing appointment ever. I had been worried about this for the past few weeks. You may be wondering what the hell it was, well here goes. I had an appointment with the colonoscopy team at 1.30pm. The name alone sends shivers up my spine and should I say up my ass. Yes the Colonoscopy is a camera up the rear to check out the colon etc. The Oncology team had seen a shadow inside the colon and decided that a colonoscopy was the best thing to have done. I was convinced up to the time of arrival in the department that this would happen today. How wrong I was and it appears I would have to relive the nightmare at a later date. It was merely an appointment to tell me that it was needed to confirm or cancel any fears that the team had. I don't think that anything is actually wrong but to please everyone I accepted the challenge to have a colonoscopy. In a way I was relieved that it was not going to happen today but then again in another way I would have liked to get it out of the way today. Now I would have to accept the challenge and go through the procedure at a later date. I was told that a letter confirming date and time of the Colonoscopy would arrive in my post in the near future. By having this procedure everyone gets to know exactly what is wrong in there or not.

Another thing that I must tell you is that I have been going through very low body temperature since 2014 after Chemo had begun. It is one of the reactions to treatment in many cancer patients. My gas and electric bills are sometimes horrendous. I also wear a hoodie a lot to keep warm so then I do look like a typical cancer patient. I have tiredness, sickness, feeling cold, peripheral neurapathy, swollen face and neck with trapped fluid, foot cramps, body shocks. These problems are easing now occasionally but the cold body and lymphodema etc do remain. I still, of course, have this feed tube in my abdomen into my stomach and I suppose I have got accustomed to the cold body but it is annoying for family and friends when they come to visit or stay and the temperatures in the house are tropical throughout the year and I am still shivering cold in a hoodie. Ask any cancer patient and the cold and fatigue is the common problem in all of us. As my condition is terminal, you could say that I in fact are part of a "dying breed". If I haven't mentioned it up to now, for past couple of years, cold body is a persistent problem. Okay, moving on and I didn't have long to wait for that colonoscopy appointment letter to arrive in the post. The big day is today on Saturday June 10th at 2.40pm. I really did not expect a Saturday appointment. I was of course fasting since last night in view of the fact where the camera is going to be put into. This was going to be my most awful experience but it had to be done to put everyone's mind at ease. Once it is done then everything else can then move on. Right now a bowel movement is the first to move on. Gaz was with me and stayed in the waiting room. I signed the consent form and gave them my medical list of tablets etc. I literally signed a consent for someone unknown to me to shove a camera up my ass. I entered another smaller waiting room with a cubicle attached to that. I put on a gown which was open at the back for obvious reasons and left all my clothes in the cubicle. Each patient had their own separate area. A couple of nurses were there with other patients but we all knew that we were there for only one particular reason, yes we were all about to have a camera inserted up our bums. It had to be done. No going back now. I could hear the other patients being asked to leave the comfort of the cubicle etc and have the procedure done. Within a couple of minutes a nurse and another male person in medical scrubs came into my area and asked a few questions. The male on scrubs was Dr I. N. This medical man was just so, so good at his work. Before I knew it he asked me questions about if I had fasted correctly etc. He told me what was involved and how quick it would be. He put me at ease. I signed another form and then I realised that this hunk was going to be the one inserting the camera up my ass. If anyone had seen us as we both walked away in the direction of the room where it was all going to happen. It must have looked strange from behind as this male led me in a gown away to face the music. I followed his instructions as I climbed up on this table type trolley. The gown that I wore was worn with the back open and therefore accessible. I followed his instructions and to be honest I really do not know why the nurse was with me. Picture the scene with this pretty nurse standing beside me holding my hand as this guy doing the colonoscopy on me was about to do his work with this tube with a camera on its tip. As the nurse held my right hand I can't help thinking that I was glad that the camera holder and my hand holder had the correct jobs on hand. I was lying on my side and naked from the waist down, a charming view no doubt. If the camera was about to cause pain then holding my hand would actually help. I was on my side and the gown was lifted. My butt was exposed and I was asked to bring my knees up towards my chin. I assume gel was on the tip of the camera because there was absolutely no pain at all, not even uncomfortable. Don't get me wrong. I knew the camera was already up in there doing its looking around etc but after a few minutes this medical guy calling the shots told me that it was all over. After that the hand holding stopped. I was grateful that she was there to put me at ease in the first place. After the excess gel etc was wiped away, pardon the image, I was asked by the Doctor N to return to my cubicle and get dressed after which he would then come to me and have a chat. The nurse said her goodbye and she walked away to hold another hand and put someone else at ease. Both of them were excellent and I'm certain my day would have been far worse without them. I got dressed and my day was going to get better. The camera operator returned and told me that all was clear in there and there were no problems to be seen. I guessed that all along but had to be sure about it. I left the area after thanking him and shook the hand that earlier had guided a soft tipped camera up my ass. I will say one thing though. I was stupid to have been worried over nothing. It must be the same as checking for prostate cancer and was over before I knew about it. I returned to Gaz in the waiting room. All was okay, no walking funny or anything like that at all. I will however be requesting a cushion for the next few days every time I rest my ass. I will not forget this day ever and life goes on as best as I can make of it. I suppose what I do mean is that if anybody is facing a similar type of invasive procedure, have no worries as there is nothing to be worried about and it's best to get it checked out. They have seen it all before.

——— # # # ———

SATURDAY JUNE 24th 2017. I drove to London Standstead Airport and flew to Dubrovnik in Croatia for a short holiday of seven days which is enough that my system can handle at this time. At least I am able to travel and have a break from it all. Gaz and his girlfriend are already out in the region on holiday and will meet up with me tonight and then, after our holiday, come home together. I arrived early in the day and got settled in the apartment that we had earlier booked under AirBnB. I found it very hot but I need some sun and vitamin D in me. Then I may not look so sick from the cancer and the awful treatment. Later that evening I walked down to nearby shops etc and waited before Gaz arrived by taxi to meet me on a street corner. Over the next few days, I hired a car and from then on we went everywhere by car. We visited beaches and even drove down to Montenegro for a day. I loved the holiday and enjoyed being with the the people that are my closest. Whatever happens from now on at least I had time with Gaz. That boy is part of me and I can honestly say I would give my life for him at a moments notice. I suppose any parent would do the same but Gaz, let me tell you now, that I love you with all my heart whenever or whatever happens. On Saturday July 1st we arrived home from Croatia into Standstead Airport. We were delayed by 1.5 hours leaving Dubrovnik all because someone miscounted. We had an extra bag in the hold of plane with no owner. It turned out that it belonged to a child and the mix up escalated from there. Eventually we took off after another passenger somehow pointed out the error. We then discovered it was her child and her fault.

Our holiday was over and we were to continue with our lives and in my case battling this f*****g cancer. Now that I got a bit of a suntan I don't look so sickly. On Friday July 7th at 1.30pm, I had an appointment with Yvonne my CHANT dietican at St Christopher's clinic in Orpington. It was basically to check on my progress and to log my eating in all aspects like what I eat and when I eat. She is happy with me and what I am doing in the circumstances. On Saturday 8th July, my brother Liam arrived to visit me. It was great seeing him again. We had a good catch up and he left again on Sunday. The next morning was Monday 10th and I had a PET Scan in St Thomas's Hospital. No need for me to explain this procedure, I have become a near expert on these procedures now. The scan was at 10am and I was out of there by 1.20pm. I got the hospital transport home and took it easy for the remainder of the day. Daytime telly is good. On today Tuesday 18th I am shitting myself with fear and torment for tomorrow. The worry in me now is so so much and I have no idea how to control it. Why? Tomorrow I get my Scan results from Theresa or one of the team. Wednesday July 19th, I had the appointment for 1.30pm and I was seen at about 2.30pm. It was Andriana, one of her team that I saw. She told me that there was increased progression in the cancer in both my right lung and windpipe. To treat it she is going to introduce a chemotherapy drug called Docetaxel and possible introduction to a trial drug. Either way, further treatment is due soon to treat the cancer. I was with Gaz of at the meeting and we left there quietly. Inside I was devastated. I did not expect to hear the news in that room but that's how my cancer story is going, one day up and the next day down. I do not have a lot to write now at the moment from. Compare this to the early stages of my cancer when every day something different happened and now look at today, for example, when my sickness outside has levelled out and I do not have a lot to say. This just shows that I feel good overall and no crazy stuff is happening to me. Inside as we know from the last scan, things are different and the cancers are growing.

On August 9th I had another appointment in Oncology to sign up and receive info on the Docetaxel. Here we go again then, more chemo and what it can do to me. It scares me a little what may be about to happen or not. I signed up for 6 cycles or 18 weeks of this Docetaxel treatment. I need all the prayers in the world and it scares me. I left there and got transport home. In a way I am shocked but here goes and let's see. Thursday 10th August 2017 I had an appointment in the PRUH with Starr, re my gastric band. My weight is now 75.4 kilos. On Friday 11th I had a phone call to say my chemo treatment of Docetaxel would begin on August 23rd at 11am but on the previous day I had to attend Guys Oncology outpatient to have a pre-treatment consultation at 10am.

On Thursday August 17th, I attended in Keston the passing out ceremony of Jamie my friend a police dog handler and his dog Blake. A great experience it was. That evening at home I got a puncture in my new car and then the worst thing in a long time happened, my feed tube (the Rig) got blocked. I went to A and E and after a long wait, I was told to go home as nobody was available to sort it and I should come back tomorrow but someone would call first. This is a disgrace to send me home like that and expect a call from a doctor. Needless to say, nobody called and I called them to be told that I should go immediately to the Ambulatory Unit in the PRUH. I went there and after a 4 hour wait was told that because the procedure was done in Guys which was a different trust then they wouldn't touch it so I was sent home again. I am totally dependent on that feed tube and now I don't know what to do.

On Monday 21st, Bromley Social Services on district nurse advice called and measured up to fit a handrail on stairs. They were also told to put me down for a high back chair. The chair was because of a recommendation from my physio Sam of the CHANT team. On the 22nd I had my pre treatment consultation at 10am in Guys. I done it before so most of it was procedure for me. Then on the big day August 23rd my latest new chemotherapy treatment begins. I feel exactly how I felt back on January 9th 2014, the day of my first ever treatment of that chemo of Cisplatin, 5FU and Cetuximab. I often think back to that day and how it started and what it done to me. I can never forget what happened then. So today brings a mix of anxiety and fear as to what will happen to me with a new drug. This one is called Docetaxel. It is only one drug so I'm hoping it will not be as toxic. The same method was used, infusion, but a lot has happened since that day. New things have been discovered since then but of course many people have failed to respond and have passed away. Now this is latest treatment for me. I attended at 11am and when asked, I approached my designated lounger and waited for the nurse to prepare and connect me up to the Infusion machine in this New Cancer Centre in Guys. The entire procedure went without any problems and when it finished I had another appointment at 2pm to have a tubogram which was to check on my feed tube (RIG). I knew it was either blocked or out of its track and the tubogram would tell this. The community dietician had organised this procedure as it had gone on for far too long now and as I was unable to eat and drink normally and the tube not working then ultimately I was getting weaker and dehydrated more and more. My RIG was replaced by a new one with a small cage to keep it in place. Lets see how this goes and if it's so good at doing its job. For days now I have suffered with a sore throat and getting dehydrated. The procedure seems to have worked. I was discharged but was very, very sick. I could feel my health going downhill so quickly but I was at home and went to bed to rest. Sunday August 27th 2017. I am now very sick and to be honest I can see myself going into hospital voluntarily. I have no intention of getting to the point where I might die alone at home. I have previously been in this position and let it go too far to the point of near death, not anymore! But, how on earth did this happen all over again. I suppose I know but it annoys me that it is happening again.

——— # # # ———

MONDAY 28th AUGUST. I feel extremely sick. I am only a matter of hours away from admitting myself into hospital. Surely this Docetaxel is not the cause of this, but it appears it is. It is just one dose in and look at what it has done to me. I just cannot understand it or believe it. What do I do now if this is the only chemo available to me. Is my body refusing to tolerate any type of chemo, surely not. I'm scared now. Tuesday 29th and I can't take anymore. I can die here if I do nothing so it's time to call the ambulance. The time is around 7pm. I told B my next door neighbour and as I already had a bag packed and ready, I was all ready to go as soon as the ambulance arrived. B came in and looked after me until then. I was able to get the house alarmed and locked up. I was carried by chair all wrapped up into the ambulance. My condition was assessed in the back of the ambulance and off we went to the PRUH. I was admitted to A and E and was there for most of the night. I am in a bad way and seriously dehydrated. They started connecting me up to bags and bags of liquid to try to get me back to normal. I was moved to AEU for another day and eventually into the Chartwell Unit in the PRUH. This is the place for those with cancer but also the seriously ill. I cannot describe it but I am very very sick and my condition is not improving at all. I am, however, soon realising that my feed tube will not be touched by anybody here in the PRUH soon. It is still in place because if it is out the hole left behind then this hole will seal itself up in 4 hours and that is a whole new ballgame all over again. Therefore the tube must be left in place unless there is an immediate replacement for it there and then. The days went by and my condition is not improving at all. Dr Barker and Dr Huq are both very concerned for me because no matter what they try, nothing is working. Fu****g politics is killing me slowly. This hospital and those I just mentioned are refusing to touch my tube or even replace it because it was done by a different hospital of a different Hospital Trust. The PRUH is Kings Trust whereas Guys, who done it originally, is part of Guys and St Thomas' Trust so that is why. If I die because of this there will be hell to pay. Can you imagine, the cancer will not kill me but an argument between hospitals might. I must tell you however that they are feeding me via TPN, which is liquid feed via a PICC line which they fitted to me. Now some type of food is getting into me and all medication is crushed and I slowly swallow it. A lot of my pain relief is by injection but it is not enough. I lie here crying, lonely and thinking the worst of what will happen to me in this hell hole of a hospital. I am confined to bed 24/7. I hate my life and I hate how I am being treated. These people better do something soon before it becomes serious. I came here on the 29th August 2017 and it is now September 4th 2017 and my blood pressure is now very low today. I was also approached by one of the staff nurses who said that a doctor wanted a serious discussion with me. It was the on call registrar who told me that my condition had got very serious and my blood pressure was dangerously low. Then the bombshell. He told me that I had Sepsis. They told me that if I got any worse and if I had a cardiac arrest, they would not get me back. I then had "DO NOT RESUSCITATE" put on my file. I told him that I disagreed but was soon told that it would be hospital policy in my case not to bring me back to life because I had terminal cancer already as a pre-existing condition. I had no choice but to accept but also I pray and pray to get out of here soon. I do not want to die and most certainly do not want to die here. Can you imagine, they will fill my bed within minutes of my death, bastards, not going to happen if I can help it. My chemotherapy appointment for 13th was cancelled but finally they realised that something had to be done. On Thursday 14th I was visited at bedside by Stacey in Intervention Radiology who told me that this afternoon they would give me a new RIG. I thought, finally, maybe I will actually get out of here. Gaz and his girlfriend came to see me several times but it's a long way from his place to the hospital here, so some nights he stayed at our home which is near the hospital. The RIG was a successful procedure in that it was different inside the stomach. It is kept in place with a cage that holds it in place. The tube is pushed into the track and the RIG has a section that is pulled into place and opens up like a cage. Clever stuff really and it works. One thing that I will never forget is that every time a RIG is removed or any type of feed tube is removed, is that if it has been in the stomach for any length of time it will be blackened and sticky to touch or look at. Reason is that stomach acids will have attacked it and possibly damaged it. If the blockage is ignored, it will get worse and anything that doesn't get through it will come back up and then there is a danger of Sepsis. This Sepsis can kill a person so there you go, do not ignore any feed tube blockages. Thank God. I was given water at first and on the next morning 15th September I was fed through the new tube. It worked and I was so relieved to have everything working again. My blood pressure was now rising a little and I spent more time now out of bed. My Sepsis problem went as my condition improved. On Monday September 18th I was asked to walk up and down the corridor in the ward. One day walking and then they told me that I was being discharged tomorrow, September 19th, from Chartwell Unit. It seems too soon and I told them but no, they insisted that I go home tomorrow the 19th. Inside I am scared that it's too soon, but I'm in no position to argue with medical experts.

——— # # # ———

Today, TUESDAY the 19th September, I am finally going home. Tonight I will be in my own bed, my own home. Ian my neighbour opposite picked me up from the hospital and took me home. I am slow to walk as I spent a lot of time in bed in the PRUH, but, I still think I came home too soon. It is still early in the day just after 3pm and I feel very weak so may go for a lie down on my bed. I put some clothes in the washing machine and put a wash on. Next on the list was preparing a new packed bag. I've been caught out before so I'm taking no chances even though I'm only out of hospital since this afternoon and everything seems to be working. One other good thing is that I am here at home alone and nobody is telling me that if I have a cardiac arrest, they will not bring me back to life. Anyhow I think it's time for a lie down. I may fall asleep so I set the alarm after locking all doors with my new security locks. Up the stairs very slowly with my stiff legs and lay on the bed. I had taken some pain relief so I soon found myself drifting off to sleep. I'm in my own bed so am gonna enjoy this lie down and sleep if I can. I woke up a couple of hours later, still tired and decided to go downstairs and have a cuppa tea. I rolled sideways out of the bed. I stood up and pulled the curtains aside and looked out the window. The time was about 6pm or a little after. I closed the curtains again and moved forward slowly. Then it happened. I moved forward and at the end of the bed, I turned sideways and lost my balance. I felt dizzy and fell down catching my back on a door knob of one of the built in wardrobes. I lost my voice and could not move with pain. I screamed in agony, that's if you can call it screaming. A really sharp pain-induced noise came out of my mouth. Yes, that is exactly as it was. It was more a noise than a voice. I was winded and thought I was going to die. I had never, ever in my life, been in a position like this. I was scared as to how I was going to get out of this. I couldn't get up but I knew I was in big trouble. I had to call an ambulance but everything was against me. I was on my bedroom floor, I couldn't stand or walk, my back was in agony and I couldn't talk. How the hell was I going to call an ambulance. All downstairs doors were locked and all security locks were on all the doors. The alarm was armed but I knew that I had to get downstairs and unlock and disable the alarm. If I called an ambulance now, they would smash the door down to get to me. My plan was to somehow get downstairs, and after opening all locks etc, I would then call Ian and Anne my great neighbours across the road from me. I had my already prepared bag here on the bed and I crawled along the floor of the bedroom slowly but in absolute agony. I realised that I had broken something in my back area of my body. I was in deep shit here but I had to get downstairs. I crawled towards the top step of the stairs and slowly step-by-step I began my pain-filled journey downstairs. It was going to take a long time. I began my slow crawl to get downstairs at about 6.40pm and this voice that was a weak noise coming from me was getting weaker and weaker. It was going to be agony moving from step to step. The time from the end of the bed to the first step was after taking just under 30 mins. It was about 7.10pm now. I eventually got downstairs at about

7.50pm. It had taken me about one hour and ten minutes to get downstairs. I managed to use the radiator to pull myself up and I used the alarm fob to disable the alarms. I got the front door opened and I called Ian my neighbour opposite on his mobile. They were great and came across and took over my care. Ian got pain relief into me and he called the ambulance. The ambulance arrived reasonably quick and sorted me out. I called Gaz and I felt sorry for him because his dad was only out of hospital a few hours and was going back in there again. I was taken into the ambulance to be stabilised before being taken away to the PRUH again. Ian and Anne secured the house, alarmed it and gave me the keys and put the alarm fob into my rucksack. I was given some gas and air as my back pain was awful. The ambulance moved off and I was on my way back to the PRUH. I then cried simply because I didn't know if I would ever see my home again. I dreaded this moment as it was happening. At least one good thing was that my feed tube was in good working order. We got to A and E and my trolley and I was wheeled into a cubicle. The gas and air was wearing off so I was given some morphine. I was checked over again and was taken after a few hours into AEU. I'm not gonna beat around the bush here but soon I had a doctor with me and he pulled the curtains. He told me that an x ray was going to be done but it was looking likely that I had broken my back. I had the x Ray and yes I had broken a bone in L1 and it was gonna be painful. I knew then what was coming next. Yes, the lecture on D N R. Yes they would not get me back if I had a cardiac arrest etc. I had to say yes as these people were adamant about it. Can you imagine being told so often about not getting me back. They certainly got their message across. On Saturday 23rd I had an X ray, I was moved into Surgical 7 and the hard recovery struggle back started. I was confined to bed and was now getting used to wearing a body brace which they insisted I wear most of the time. I was still confined to bed, no movement and nurses giving me bed baths etc. My blood pressure was still low as it always is.

On the 28th I was moved into Room 252 in Surgical 7, their choice not mine. I was then taken to Kings for a scan on my spine and returned same day. I was told that there was a virus on the ward and moving me to a side room was to protect me. It was looking very likely that my 60th Birthday would be in the PRUH. I felt awfully sick and in terrible pain. My back was killing me and I thought I would never get out of here.

On Sunday October 1st I was told that I had an infection in my chest. I do not need a chest infection in here and then I was told that all visitors would wear face masks and gowns or aprons. I looked like I was after contracting Ebola. Can you imagine the scene. Every time I had visitors, I didn't recognise some of them until they were right hanging over me because of all the gear that they were wearing. Funny really but right now my immune system is low and I can easily catch this vomiting bug that's in the whole hospital.

On Wednesday October 4th, I had a lovely surprise as the room door slowly

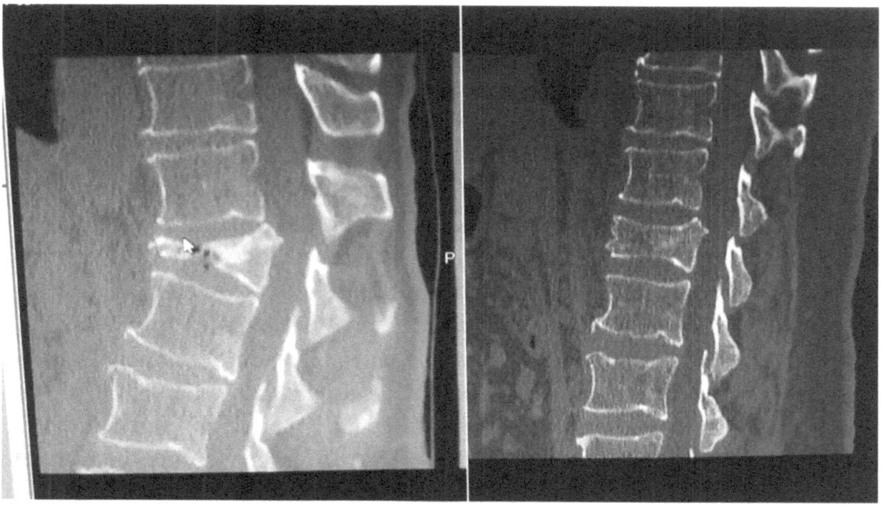

My broken back.

opened and this figure covered in plastic apron etc came in the door to me. My sister Mary had come all the way from Ireland on her own to visit me with balloons etc for my birthday. It was difficult for her doing all this on her own but she did it. It was truly a lovely surprise doing it all on her own for the first time. She returned home the next day but it was great to see her.

Saturday October 7th was a low key event for my 60th birthday. In the morning 5 nurses came into my room singing Happy Birthday, What a nice gesture for them to do that for me. Gaz an his girlfriend, who had been popping into see me every couple of days now, spent the whole day with me today. There were more birthday cards than usual for me. Maybe it's because I am in hospital and 60 is a big number. I was also given a walking stick today, nice birthday present, and was told that some alterations were to be done at home. Gaz had arranged to be at home with keys to let in people to give me a new stairs handrail, commode, raised toilet seat and a seat for the kitchen. They also gave me a large cushion for my back when sitting down. I lost a lot of weight while in here in hospital. I am now 63 kilos. I was 72 kilos coming in here the first time on August 29th.

Anyhow, today is October 10th and am out of bed and with help from physio. While here in hospital my pain relief is Morphine granules, 80 mgs every 12 hours and then liquid morphine as a top up when needed. I am walking up and down the corridor in Surgical 7. No more gowns and masks etc, the infection scare is over both in me and in the hospital. It looks like I am on the mend and going home soon. Over the next few days the physios had me walking with a stick and then up and down stairs.

On Friday 13th I was finally discharged but this time I have been walking for days so it is not too soon to go home. I was going to live to fight another day. Ian was to pick me up but Hospital insisted that hospital transport took me home. That night about 7pm they took me home. No medication and I was told it would follow later . Finally, I was eventually home. In the hospital transport on the short journey home, I shared it with 2 elderly women. As the ambulance pulled up outside my door after a five minute trip from the hospital, one of these fu****g nosey women said to the other as I struggled to walk with a stick "he could have walked, couldn't he". I turned around and said to her "Listen you two Gossipfuc***s, you both stink of stale piss and shit. I broke my back and you two will live longer than me because I also have terminal cancer". Their silence was deafening as I put them in their place. Some people are so nasty, yet it's the nasty people like them that live longer than others and therefore as a direct result, pollute and make the lives of nice people into hell. Anyhow, I went indoors and sat down to recollect what has happened over the past few weeks. It has been mad but I'm still here and my fight goes on. At about 9pm a nursing assistant on way home dropped off my medication.

On the 14th my boiler packed in. The part that has the switch to control the heating and water has malfunctioned. I called out Home Rescue 24/7 to sort it out but had to pay £35 in advance. They said it would take up to 10 days to come out to repair it. My friend Mary the plumber dropped me off an electric Halogen heater. On the 14th and 15th I had carers coming in but after two days they said that I no longer needed help as I was okay to do things for myself.

On Monday 16th I had a visit from a physio at 11am and at 4pm a visit by a nurse from St Christopher's. While I was in the PRUH, I had been put in contact with St Christopher's. They are also doing house contact visits to anyone with cancer. No need to go to their hospice while I am still okay to have them come to me at home. It was a great visit and many concerns of mine were resolved. I was assured that they would help me in any way possible. They took on board the fact that my pain relief is sometimes delayed in getting to me. I am confident that this issue will be sorted sooner rather than later.

On Tuesday October 17th a district nurse came to me at 4pm. I am, however, getting better being at home. The hospital was great to get me back to health but I do not want to go back there at anytime soon. District nurse due again on 20th.

On Friday 20th Hannah my CNS from Guys Oncology came to see me at home at 10.15am. I realise that my DOCETAXEL treatment may be back soon unless something else is on the cards. One dose of DOCETAXEL was all I had before I ended up in hospital for the first time ages ago. The district nurse also came on the 20th at 4pm.

On Saturday 21st, I with Gaz and his girlfriend went to the O2 to see Micky Flanagan. The staff there were fantastic and on arriving there they took me in a wheelchair to my seat and afterwards came to my seat to take me to the area where our taxi was due to pick us up. We had a great night and I am thankful that I was there. A few weeks ago it was all looking like it wasn't going to happen but it did. Fantastic. I feel tired but that's to be expected as my condition recovers. On 23rd a heating engineer came out and only looked at the boiler before leaving again. They wanted £90 but I refused. He left empty handed. No work was done. I stood my ground and continued to refuse to pay anything to them. District nurse came on the 24th.

On the 28th and 29th I felt very sick, another chest infection. District nurse requested antibiotics from my doctor when she came on 28th. The antibiotics came on 30th by chemist delivery. Ever since I was discharged my pain relief was Morphine liquid and also Morphine granules.

On the 30th a doctor from St Christopher's came out to me when I asked for a home visit from him. He immediately increased my Morphine granules from 80 every 12 hours to 130 every 12 hours. He contacted my GP surgery and advised the same. That was a big help to control my pain. I also signed up today for online Sainsburys home delivery. I will only use it up until I can again get out to do my shopping normally.

Tuesday October 31st 2017 was trick or treat night. Loads of kids in the street tonight with parents. It is little things like this that I thought I would never see again. That night I dimmed the lights and watched telly and for no reason I burst out crying. I say no reason but in fact, there is one big reason. It is the actual relief that I am home and still alive and came so close to actually passing away again this time. Since the day I was diagnosed in 2013. I take nothing for granted. Ever since the day I was born and this applies to every person or living thing. Since the day I was born I am actually dying as is every living thing. In my case however the medical people have told me that my cancer is going to cause me to die before those living normally. Life certainly is shit!

——— # # # ———

WEDNESDAY NOVEMBER 1st 2017. I have an 1pm appointment in Guys to see Theresa or one of the team. It was Theresa herself and she said that the scan showed that there was no cancer in my bones which was the scare after I fell. She is glad that St Christopher's are on board to modify my medications. Theresa also told me that she was considering now to put me on IMMUNOTHERAPY treatment as a clinical study and as a means of eventually controlling my cancer. I am very excited about this prospect happening and Theresa is happy to make inroads into its implementation fighting my cancer. She also said that I would be under the responsibility of Dr Bell in Kings College Hospital as regards my fall and my back injury which would take quite a while to recover from. On the 2nd November I had a quote at 4pm to clean my carpets for £135. On 3rd my boiler problem was sorted. Great, heat and hot water again. In the afternoon I had a visit from a district nurse and Jo from St Christopher's. Jo was a senior nurse. On the 6th, I had 2 cleaners to blitz clean my house top to bottom. All the time in hospital means a lot of dust has settled. They sorted it out after a few hours. On the 7th, Nutricia collected old Fortisip and on 8th they delivered new Nutricia Fortisip. My back is very painful and will be for a long time yet, maybe even years. I curse the day that I fell in my bedroom. On November 13th I had a PET Scan in St Thomas's Hospital at 11.45am. It took me all f*****g day to get home in the hospital transport. All around the houses seeing different parts of London and its surroundings. I got indoors at 8pm. My pain relief is now running low so I have to ration it until I get a delivery tomorrow (Tuesday). I asked St Christopher's to send out a doctor to review my pain which is getting worse. On Friday 17th a doctor from St Christopher's came out to me and sorted out all my pain relief. A district nurse also came out and changed my RIG dressings.

——— # # # ———

SATURDAY 18th. I feel bad and in a lot of pain. The pain continued for days and days. On the 21st I had a ZOLLENTRONIC infusion in the PRUH at 2pm. I was wiped out after it. On the 22nd I had an appointment in Guys about the Immunotherapy trial. On the 23rd I had all my carpets cleaned throughout and at 11.30am and on the 28th I had an appointment with my dentist. All went well and that my friends and readers is the end of November and what a f*****g shit month it was. Bring on December.

——— # # # ———

FRIDAY DECEMBER 1st 2017 my stomach feels sore to touch and I think it may be my bloody RIG tube playing up. More problems and Christmas is only weeks away. Saturday 2nd December and my tube is leaking I feel so low now and this can only mean that the tube is blocked at the stomach end. When I say leaking, I mean the liquid going in and that includes Morphine but Fortisip drinks are not getting through and are leaking through the dressings.

On 5th the tube got unblocked somehow and I have no idea how. Sometimes it is how I stand or lie at an angle. Sometimes it is luck but I fear something is wrong because it is still sore in my stomach. One thing that needs explaining is how the tube gets blocked up. The part of the tube that enters into the stomach is constantly being attacked by stomach acids, so as a result the tube is classed as alien to it. I cannot remember if I told you this before or not. Anyhow, inside the stomach some tissue grows onto the tip and around

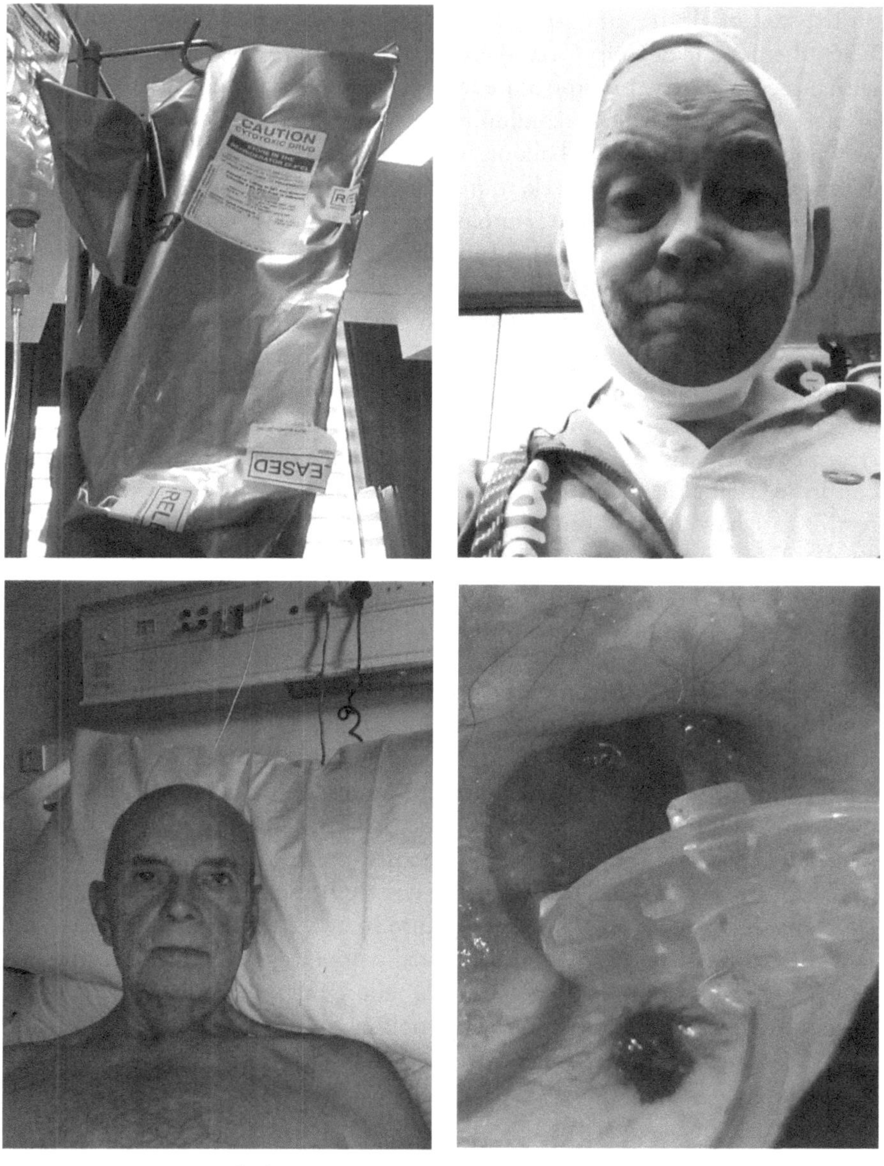

My treatment packs hanging up ... My face swelling from fluid retention ... my feed tube infection in stomach

the tube inside the stomach area. In an attempt to make it difficult for this to happen, every day or so I have to rotate the tube to knock off any tissue attempting to grow onto it. It sometimes works but when it doesn't then it's time for a trip to the A and E. Also, inside the tube itself stomach fluids grow on the wall of all the tube so to deter that, it is advised to flush it with Soda Water. Lemonade or Coca Cola is not advised at all. My tube is secured in place with a cage type structure to secure it in place but some RIG units are secured in place by a small balloon containing 3mls of water. The cage version is not very popular as I prefer the balloon with the 3mls of water to keep it in place. This is changed once every week, more than likely on a Friday. So now you know my friends. Anyhow the tube is unblocked for now so we carry on using it.

On Tuesday 5th, I had a dental appointment and all is well. On Wednesday 6th I had an appointment with Theresa or the team in Oncology in Guys. It was a great meeting as it was decided that the trial drug and associated biopsies were too damaging to me but that the Immunotherapy drug that we spoke about before, called NIVOLUMAB, is probably the best for me. There are no associated Biopsies and it was all systems go. Immunotherapy is to be my future treatment so I was more than happy to sign the consent forms. It was then confirmed that treatment would start after Christmas. I am so looking forward to this as I have heard so much about Immunotherapy and it has had good results. This Nivolumab was on a list of trial drugs but it has had good success results and the Government has licenced it to be used across the system. It's great news all around as it will replace the toxic sickness linked to Chemotherapy. This "Nivolumab" Immunotherapy basically works like this. The cancer has tricked my immune system or any immune system into thinking it's okay, so the cancer carries on and it doesn't give a shit as nothing is fighting it apart from Chemotherapy or Radiotherapy. These treatments kill all the cells, good and bad. However, now we have Immunotherapy in many named drugs. One of them is my one called "NIVOLUMAB" and it lights up the cancer and makes it exposed for all its badness. It boosts my Immune system which then fights the cancer. Basically my own body is fighting the cancer and the side effects are less, much less. That is the planm so now I can enjoy Christmas, but first there is this RIG problem to be sorted before it gets too bad. On the 7th, I took two suits and 3 trousers to a local tailor, Tailor Arif is the name of the business and I used them before. They took in all the trousers and all the suits for just over £240. That is much cheaper than buying new clothes, new suits or new trousers.

On the 9th of December my tube is blocked again. I called Rosie my dietician who referred me to the PRUH tomorrow 10th to have it sorted. On the 10th I went into the PRUH and Intervention Radiology to see Stacey. They did something to it and it was clear again.

On the 11th, I had my Christmas lights put up in the guttering by my window cleaner. Over the next couple of days I was in and out of the PRUH like a yo-yo as my tube was playing up so much. On the 15th we all attended the Panto in Bromley. It was a really great night. On the 18th I had an appointment with Karen in St Christopher's clinic as regards any problems. All is well and it is so good to have these meetings to get things sorted out before they get out of hand. On 19th I saw my dentist, all is well but on the 20th, five days before Christmas, the feed tube is again playing up. I called Rosie my Dietician and she called Stacey in the PRUH Intervention Radiology. Stacey called me and asked me to go in the next day, the 21st at 10.30am. I went there next morning and they did something to it again but said it would have to be changed completely in 2018. At least it was sorted for Christmas. I cannot thank Rosie and Stacey enough for sorting it out at such short notice and saving my Christmas. One thing I forgot to mention is that, with the tube, it is in a track of flesh from outside in the abdomen into the stomach and if it comes out of its track, the track has to be filled by a new tube or a plastic rod within 4 hours otherwise that track space fills up and the tissue heals up like an earing that comes out of its pierced space.

On Sunday 24th I drove to Farnham and Garreth's girlfriend's family. Gaz and I were invited to spend Christmas there. We all had a lovely Christmas and I came back home on the 27th. Gaz was with me for the next few days at home.

On December 31st, I spent it at home alone to recall all my life and it's happenings during 2017. Just after 11.30pm Gaz called me and wished me a happy new year. He was seeing in the New year with his girlfriend in their own home. I saw in the New Year and my recollections of 2017 carried on well into 2018. I went over everything in my mind. I was even thinking about my diaries and how this book was being put together. I don't have much more to add tonight to this part of the book but it doesn't end here. As it is well past midnight and it's into 2018, all I have to say is Happy New Year 2018 and I will write again in a few hours where it will definitely be 2018. Goodnight.

——— # # # ———

Good Morning all it's 10am MONDAY JANUARY 1st 2018 and I am welcoming in the New Year 2018 with a chest infection, however, I had a phone call from Stacey in the PRUH Intervention Radiology. She wants me to attend in her Department tomorrow morning, Tuesday January 2nd, where the rig is to be changed to a new one with a balloon to hold it in place inside the stomach. Great, this is the best news as the balloon is more favourable to me than the cage. Anyhow let's get things moving. Everything is happening all of a sudden. I have this nasty chest infection, tube being replaced and my 1st treatment day of Immunotherapy is on Wednesday 3rd January but I expect it to be changed now because of my chest infection.

——— # # # ———

Morning all. Today is January 2nd and I am at the PRUH in Intervention

Radiology. Stacey got me to sign the consent forms and I changed into a gown before walking into the procedure room. I will not be walking out of here. I had to get on a step and onto a trolley. I was prepared for the procedure and had my belly area exposed. I was awake for it all, I just had the abdomen cleaned with Iodine. I had the area injected with local anaesthetic and it all began. The doctor in charge got out a box with a new feed tube with balloon fitting at the tip which was to be inside the stomach. As the track was already there, the doctor collapsed the cage in the old tube. As expected I saw it being pulled out. I was wide awake and it was black and sticky with tissue and stomach acids on it from where it had been for the past number of months. It made a small "pop" sound as it came out. He then simply put it in a clinical waste bin and forced the new one into the track of the old one. All done and it was complete and thorough. I simply got down from my trolley and returned to the cubicle and got dressed. The numbness soon wore off and my stomach was a little sore from being tugged and pulled about. It actually felt like it did before and similar to being kicked in the stomach. My good neighbour Ian, collected me from the hospital. I was waiting outside the main entrance and as people walked about, I bet nobody guessed that 30 minutes earlier I was on a trolley and had a stomach procedure done. It was all amazing really. Ian picked me up and took me home. I rested for the remainder of the day. Tomorrow is my first Immunotherapy treatment day. My chest was bad and I had to tell them in Guys. They immediately cancelled my treatment so I then had to cancel the hospital transport that was picking me up. Over the next few days my chest infection took hold and it terrified me that I might have to go back into hospital. Fortisip saved me and I kept my strength up. My district nurse contacted my GP and he sent me out a course of antibiotics. I was extremely tired but soon I was on the mend. On the 10th January I attended Guys Oncology at 1.30pm. I saw Adriana. She also noticed that my weight had dropped considerably. I told her that it was because of my chest infection to which she agreed. She did notice however that despite the weight loss, I was better than expected and treatment would go ahead as usual on January 19th. At last I have a date that "Nivolumab" would be given to me by infusion at 3pm. That really was the whole point of the meeting but, before I left Guys, I had to have my height and weight taken, Then one more thing was to have a blood test. If the blood was okay then treatment would go ahead as planned on January 19th.

Okay, back to today and it's January 12th and Bromley Council are collecting, as arranged, my sharps bin. As you know and I am quite used to it now, every night I inject myself with Clexane 100 mgs. It also has another name called Enoxaparin. My belly is badly bruised now. I have been injecting myself now for quite a long time but I have to inject in alternative sides of my belly otherwise the bruising gets far worse . My sharps bin was collected around 11am and they gave me 2 more in its place. I am very tired and my body feels cold. I wonder what I'll be like on the 19th which is treatment day.

——— # # # ———

GOOD MORNING FRIDAY JANUARY 19th and it's treatment day. I am hugely excited as this day could be the start of a turnaround in my condition. If it works, then it will give me more time to live and delay the inevitable. I got the hospital transport as usual and, to be honest, I really didn't care if it was late getting there or not. On arrival at the New Cancer Centre I made my way to the treatment suite which is in the same place as Chemotherapy. I was called in after I handed over my appointment card at the reception desk. I would get it later after treatment with the time and date of the next appointment here. I was called into the treatment suite B which is one of 4 different suites. I had a canula inserted into my left arm and within minutes the machine pumping the flushing of the line into the canuala begins. After 30 mins or so the pack of clear liquid NIVOLUMAB was connected up to the same pumping machine. I could have just watched the clear liquid drip in slowly into me but instead I just lay back in my recliner. The tea lady came around and I had a tea and a sandwich. After having that I soon nodded off to sleep. I woke up as the end of my treatment was happening. I was stiff but otherwise okay. After a while I then made my way to the nurses station desk but a nurse came towards me with my blue appointment card. My next appointment would be February 2nd 2018. I was all excited. I now knew that I was walking around with a revolutionary type of treatment going around inside me and getting to all areas of my body. Maybe there were other people here with the same stuff running around in their veins but I was feeling greedy now and this was my moment to probably have a sneaky internal moment of silent grinning and knowing that I had stuff in me that may actually give me extra time. God Bless the NHS. I left the suite at about 4.50pm and made my way downstairs to the transport lounge. Michelle and Maria are both on today. There I gave my details to Michelle who entered my name into the system and I awaited my transport home. Transport arrived reasonably quick at about 5.35pm and I was home by 6.50pm. On Monday 22nd I had an appointment with Karen Davies in St Christopher's at 2pm. She measured my height and took my weight. I then discovered that I had lost 2 inches of my height because of my back being broken last year when I broke a bone and everything collapsed downwards. I left the room but apart from my height news, I was reasonably pleased. My weight was 64.5 kilos. It was then I remembered back in the days when I was overweight and was 146 kilos. What a difference now.

Tuesday 23rd I had a 10.45am dental appointment and on Friday 25th I had an appointment at 3.40pm with Mr Bell or a member of his team. I had a scan and within minutes was told that Mr Bell was happy with my back etc and I was told that I didn't have to wear the body brace anymore. To be honest I stopped wearing that brace at around Christmas which was a number of weeks ago. Again, I used hospital transport to take me there and bring me home. I still have a walking stick to help me get around however.

On the 31st of January, I had an appointment at 4pm to see my consultant and had a blood test. It was basically to see if I was coping okay with the treatment. I told her exactly how I felt. I had only experienced one session of Immunotherapy and apart from being tired I was reasonably okay. My current up-to-date side effects and treatment are now as follows. I have a little Peripheral Neurapathy, extreme tiredness, the occasional but rare nose bleed, sore knees, very sore back which needs very regular pain relief of Morphine Granules, Liquid Morphine, Soluble Paracetamol, a feed tube that needs dressing every day and every day self injecting Clexane into an already heavily bruised belly. Overall it's not too bad compared to what it was not too long ago.

——— # # # ———

So now we are into February 2018 and today is FRIDAY FEBRUARY 2ND. It's my second day of NIVOLUMAB treatment of Immunotherapy. It is a very early start as hospital transport arrived to pick me up at 7am. There was already another lady in the car who also had an early treatment appointment by Radiotherapy. I arrived in Guys at 9.10am and as I already had blood taken on the Wednesday. I assumed all was okay as treatment began near enough on time at about 9.45am. Because of my early start, the nurse looking after me went to get me a cup of tea and a sandwich. She returned with tea and a cheese and ham sandwich. That sorted out the early start missing out on a cuppa. The treatment proceeded as normal. I had my cuppa and soon nodded off after they had prodded and poked me to get the canuala in the right place. I have no idea how but I woke up after about an hour and a half just as it all was reaching completion by 12 noon. I hope I didn't snore but they could have redecorated the place around me and I wouldn't have known about it one bit whatsoever. I stood up after a few minutes but I was very stiff and tired. I grabbed my walking stick and got all my bits and pieces together, mobile phone, watch, and headphones. I got my black puffer jacket and my next plan was to get into the toilet and get some Morphine pain relief into me. I never needed to do this before but I had some with me and it's just as well. I won't be home for hours yet, so happy days. In about ten minutes I had collected my next appointment time on the booklet and after saying my goodbyes to Lucy in the nurses station, I was in the lift and on my way downstairs to see Michelle or Maria in Transport and book my transport home. Michelle was there but busy on the phone so Maria arranged it. In this transport lounge waiting room, everything is so lovely and relaxed just as it should be with so many very sick people here. The girls here manning the phones contribute so much of course to the atmosphere and they seem to know every patient's name and that of their family and friends. The expected waiting time here is between 60 and 90 minutes. Today my transport took just over 90 minutes to pick me up in a patient transport ambulance. I was sharing with 5 other people and by the looks of things, no heating in the transport and a trip around south London and into Kent was on the cards. Still, never mind, I had a good day, pain relief had worked soon after I took it and I was on my way home. After all the drop offs, I reached home around 4pm. I just rested for the remainder of the day. Over the next few days I was wiped out but no sickness. I had nausea but Domperidone anti-sickness took that away.

On Wednesday 7th I had an appointment at St Christopher's in Orpington with Kate my Physio. My major problem now also apart from the cancer is my neck muscles are so weak now that my head droops forward and is not correcting itself. Kate saw how bad it was and made a report. I am hoping that I have sessions where a physio gives me proper manipulating of my neck. Nothing else works so, let's see. I am still very tired however and on the 8th I saw Starr in the PRUH just to check on my non-working gastric band. She's happy and my weight is 68.2 kilos.

On Friday 9th I am back in the St Christopher's clinic to see Yvonne my dietician and Cate my CNS from Guys at 11.15am. Everybody is happy with me. Everybody is suddenly happy with my condition. On 13th February 2018 Nutricia collected old Fortisip and delivered new stock. They also dropped off new syringes for getting Meds and food into my tube.

Friday 16th, today is 3rd session of "Nivolumab". Appointment was 8.30am with a 6am pick up from my home. It all went well with a blood test at 8.30am, then a long 2 hour wait for blood results. They were good and treatment then began at 10.50am. I got home at 4.30pm and of course the usual tiredness happened.

On Thursday 22nd, the district nurse emptied the 3mls of water in the tube in my belly. Somehow her finger caught it and the tube came out. She panicked so it was down to me. Part of the tube was attached to my belly with tape but I had to plug the hole with my little finger. Stomach acids and blood soon eased out and I then forced the tube back inside. I then held it in place and put a few mls of water into it to secure it in place. It worked and things soon returned to normal. The smell however of stomach acids and the dirty black colour shocked me, I was shocked but everything has to be done sometime for the first time. This was one of those moments for me and I survived. As you know if the tube comes out the hole must be plugged or filled within 4 hours like an earring space otherwise it seals up and then a trip to A and E. The nurse was very relieved but it surprised me that she panicked. Next time I will know if she is in my house doing my dressings. Changing the water in the tube is part of her jobs to do, it could be very nasty indeed if I hadn't done what I did. Tuesday 27th and the snow is heavy here.

Friday 28th is my appointment with Adriana in Oncology at 2.30pm and I also had a blood test this time on the Wednesday. Andriana is very happy with me and my weight is up to 71.5 kilos. Gaz was not with me today as his work was needing him. However, I guessed it would go well as this treatment is doing well for me apart from a few minor problems. These problems will be with me for a long time and I am coping with them as well. I left there knowing that a CT scan was being planned for me in the near future. I am a very happy cancer patient now. If there is such a person in this life as "a happy cancer patient". I went downstairs with a spring in my limp. My head however is annoying me being drooped forward and it as it seems to be getting worse. Apart from that it is terrible walking around with my head hanging forward and also getting around with a walking stick. Bring on my next treatment on Friday 2nd March at 9am.

——— # # # ———

Good Morning all. Today is MARCH 1st 2018 and it's Thursday and Gaz's 28th birthday. I cannot believe that Gaz, my boy, is 28 years old today. One thing that I am glad about is that even though my cancer is still there, so am I, to enjoy watching my only son grow and work. He has achieved so much in life, including buying his own property and is in a secure job. I have no worries about him but I would like to be around for a while yet and the way I feel right now, my problems are becoming, shall we say more, manageable. I couldn't see myself saying that a few months ago. I realise it could all go downhill tomorrow so for now I'm going to make the most of it all. The weather also is bad with very heavy snowfalls. I am the "snow friends" coordinator for my road. This means that the Bromley Council supply me with grit and salt for the residents on my road. I also help organise street parties in our road. It keeps me occupied and of course does writing this book based on my day-to-day entries in my diaries.

——— # # # ———

SATURDAY MARCH 3rd. The snow is finally melting and in my road so many people are planning and building for the future. Some of my neighbours are putting in new driveways in block paving. I have even looked to the future by getting a quote for a new driveway from the road into my front door. I have also asked for quotes for new bathroom suites on two levels of my house and new curtains in my bedroom.

——— # # # ———

On WEDNESDAY 7th MARCH, this is how things can suddenly go downhill overnight. This morning I have made panic phone calls to Oncology and my GP. I have been coughing up blood since I woke at 7.45am. Thick clots of blood and no idea where they're coming from. To be honest, I am worried sick. My Oncology has advised to keep an eye on it and if it carries on then to tell them and be prepared to put a bag together and go to nearest A and E. I would probably have done that anyway. It's never happened before so let's see. All throughout the day, it repeated once but a lot less. I decided to wait it out and hope for the best. It happened less and less though until Friday 10th it finally stopped. I am so happy but it shows that things can go downhill at a moment's notice.

On 11th and 12th I had a stomach upset and on Tuesday 13th that cleared up. What next! It's like the body of mine is having a shot at all the bad things to happen to me. Also today, the 13th March 2018, I saw Karen of St Christopher's in Orpington at 11am and after logging all my incidents Karen was happy with things overall. My head, however, has dropped forward more and is not improving. Parts of my soles of my feet are sometimes numb. My back is very sore and I still need loads of more Morphine to ease it. Will this back problem ever end. My walking stick is so helpful to get me around. I am still injecting blood thinning of Clexane every night and will be to the end of my life. I left Karen's clinic and went home Wednesday 14th. No blood test in Guys but on Friday 16th, I have to go in early for 9.30am. I was picked up by Hospital transport at 7am and it was going to be one hell of a busy tiring day.

——— # # # ———

Good morning. It's FRIDAY 16th MARCH 2018 and a busy day lies ahead. Transport that was due here at 7am but came late at 7.20am. There was one other person in the car and we chatted all the way to Guys. We both chatted and exchanged stories and jokes about our cancer and what we are hoping for. This other lady is in a better position than I am but, Bless her, she still has cancer and it must be hell for her and her young family to go through it. We picked up one other patient and all three of us, who never met before, got on so well. Time flew by and we got to Guys early. On arrival at the New Cancer Centre in Guys we all went our separate ways but no doubt we would meet up again soon. It's a big place but we are all in the same boat and we all want the same ending. Not all of us however will achieve our goals. I checked in electronically and it was already 9.15am. I first had a blood test at 9.30am which would take a couple of hours to get results back before my treatment. I was due to have Immunotherapy at 11.30am and Lympodema clinic at 1.45pm. After my blood test I went up to the Lympodema clinic and asked them to change my appointment to an earlier one as I had a lot of spare time on my hands. They immediately changed it to 11am. This was great. I therefore had this Lympodema clinic at 11am and then Immunotherapy at 11.30am, that's if the blood tests results are back on time before treatment. I had my 11am appointment and then went to the Chemotherapy Department to have my Immunotherapy treatment. Treatment started late at 12 noon and ended at around 2pm. The day went well and even though everything fitted into place when rearranged, it was a long day. I went downstairs when all was finished and checked into transport to go home. I got back at about 4.50pm The weekend was okay. No after effects from the treatment and on March 23rd had a C T Scan in Guys at 9.45am. I have no idea why a CT Scan as I always have a PET Scan for my cancer. My dietician appointment today at 11.15am with Yvonne in St Christopher's in Orpington was cancelled. Just as well, so I could have this scan in Guys. The scan went well. Transport there and back was good. Easter weekend was coming up but ever since I had radiotherapy, my taste buds are messed up as nowadays I don't like chocolate.

——— # # # ———

On WEDNESDAY MARCH 28th I had an appointment to see one of the team, as per usual, on Wednesdays every two weeks or so. Gaz wasn't with me as it was only a routine outpatient clinic appointment. I had arranged to text or call him later anyway if there was anything else planned in future or whatever. One of the team, Gemma, came out to see me in the waiting room and said there is a small delay. The appointment was for 2.30pm and she had just came out to me at 2.50pm. I asked her about how much longer and what she said alarmed me. She told me that some people were looking at my CT scan results and they would tell her the results when they knew more. I asked her about the CT scan and when a PET scan was happening. She then told me that they use CT scans on cancers that have treatment by Immunotherapy and that the results of my recent CT Scan would be known soon today. She then left and returned to the consultation room. I have previously had mixed news in the old consultation rooms and in these new rooms. I wished I had asked Gaz to come with me but it's too late now and it's getting late in the day. I texted him and explained what was happening. The time now is near 4pm and Claire my CNS came and sat beside me. After ten or fifteen minutes the lady in the consultation room, Gemma, came out and looked at me and made me smile. All she said was "It's good news". All of us, including Claire, went into the room and we all sat down. She then explained with a smile that as I had 2 areas of cancer in my right lung and another large area in my windpipe. Each of the 3 areas were about 8mm to 10mm. The CT scan had shown that the lung tumours had shrunk so much that they were barely visible and the windpipe one had shrunk near enough by half. I burst out crying. I couldn't believe it. All that worry over nothing. I sobbed like a baby in front of these two women. I can't believe it. I was told that this is only after 5 sessions of treatment and as agreed months ago, treatment would continue. God Bless Immunotherapy. It may be new but it works for me for now. I gathered my thoughts together and I hugged them both, sobbing a little. I left the room still tearful and outside some people looked at me. Claire was with me and we said Goodbye again. It was after 4.45pm and I went downstairs to Fola in the transport desk and booked my transport home. I called Gaz and he too could not believe it. Transport arrived at 5.30pm and I was home by 7.15pm having shared a patient transport ambulance with 3 other people who were dropped off before me. I got indoors and sat down and cried alone in my home. What a day, what a bloody great day. I had a cuppa and as I had taken pain relief on and off during the day, I took some more now before Bed.

Next morning Thursday 29th because of tomorrow being Good Friday and there being no treatment sessions happening. I was up early as transport picked me up at 8am for my 6th treatment of this wonderful life extending NIVOLUMAB immunotherapy. I had a permanent smile on my face all day. In the chemotherapy department where I am being treated, I was surrounded by other cancer patients lying around in their recliners having hope in a chemical bag of liquid pumped into them. I have no idea how long more this will give me but I think back to November 23rd 2013 when I was given only eighteen months to live and now four and a half years later, not only am I still here but I have the inner strength to carry on fighting this nasty aggressive sneaky disease called Cancer. Since yesterday, when I was told that my roller-coaster ride was going in the right direction, both Gaz and I still cannot believe it. Like previously I cannot be too complacent. Like in the past it can change overnight. Any cancer patient will tell you that while all around you everyone is jumping for joy, I being the patient am not jumping because it can change. Even the fakes (remember them!), well the fakes are getting in the act just because the fakes are all assholes anyway.

Thursday March 29th treatment went well with an 7.30am pick up for 10.30am treatment appointment. The next thing to happen now will be a CT scan in early June 2018 this year. Saturday March 31st ... because things are looking a little promising and I will not get too complacent, I am looking again for quotes for new units in toilets and bathroom ... Tuesday April 3rd, got my next scan date for June 4th. Friday April 13th blood test at 8am and after results back, I had treatment at 10am.

Monday 16th April a district nurse hurt me and made my Rig tube bleed after her gloves were too big for her and they got hooked in my rig. I complained about her.

Wednesday April 25th I saw my consultant at 3pm and she basically confirmed the scan date for June 4th. On Friday April 27th I received a second DNA kit in the post as the first one was faulty. Basically I am curious where in the world did my ancestors come from etc. Monday 30th I renewed my will just to give myself peace of mind to get my things in order. My son Gaz also did a similar test with the same people at Ancestry. com. And it does work because he got his results this morning. May was a quiet month and as you can probably tell, not a lot happened. My back and neck are causing me a lot of pain. Mediquip collected a few items to assist me when I broke my back. I never used the Commode, raised toilet seat and a raised step for getting into and out of the bath. I had an appointment with Karen of St Christopher's on Monday 21st May. I also had an appointment in Orpington Hospital to see a doctor in Outpatients. He said that because of my condition, as before, they will still not do anything but give me another appointment this time next year on May 20th 2019. My knee is killing me but I now have at least a date 12 months from now if I live that long.

On 23rd May I saw my consultant and had a blood test. My consultant is happy with me and confirmed my scan date for June 4th. She said if the results are good or better then it proved that it was a good move to do Immunotherapy and maybe control the cancer and have partial remission. I just cannot wait for June 4th and that scan.

On the 24th May, Vanessa and a few of my neighbours met in my place to put the final touches to our Street Party on June 2nd. The month finished with Immunotherapy treatment Number 10 at 9am. It went okay and after 2 hours I made my way home. Saturday June 2nd and we had our Street Party. We had a permit to close our road all day and all my neighbours came out and we all shared food and drink. We had live music and a great day with great weather to cap it all. Monday June 4th was CT scan day in St Thomas'Hospital at 12 noon. Leading up to the scan I was actually scared to do anything out of the ordinary in case it altered the result in any way. When I say about being careful, I mean that I did not eat or drink leading up to it. I got proper rest and sleep and generally being good and go by the rules of any scan. This scan is so, so important to me and my family. All will be revealed on June 20th, sixteen days of hell and torment to wait. In the meantime life goes on.

June 6th I had an appointment with Andrea who is a new Physio regarding my neck and back. My GP referred me to her. She was very good and gave me a list of new exercises to help me with my neck especially. I also think that she is going to refer me back to Mr Bell a Neurologist in Kings College Hospital.

On Friday June 8th I had more treatment at 9am. This was number eleven treatment. I had good results after number 5 treatment. Of course, the usual ones and the fakes are saying that of course this is number 11 so it has to be good. I let them get on with it. June 14th and I watched the opening ceremony of the World Cup. In 2013 I was given 18 months to live, now, nearly 5 years later, I am taking the piss out of the Cancer by defying it and being still alive, but then again treatments are happening all the time so while it may be my last World Cup, I just do not know. Anyhow, it is near the end of the show now and I have to begin to close this book soon. Let's see how it goes, maybe I may carry it on yet for a few more months but first let us get June 20th out of the way and these famous scan results. My appointment is at 3.30pm and Gaz is with me. It is an awesome important day for me and my family. I do not see Theresa my consultant anywhere today here in this New Cancer Centre. I do however see Gemma who is also on the team. She tends to be always in the position to give me good results, so let us see. Just after 3.30pm the signs were good but my nerves were on edge. Eventually after 4pm my name appeared on the screen to go to Consultation Room 3. I approached the open door and yes, Gemma was there at the desk and the feeling of anticipation for me went to that of fear. Unlike the last time she did not look directly at me. I know now that something is different to the last time. She said that, okay we had the scan and the windpipe tumour is now showing slight progression and in the right lung it is true that the two tumours are still spots like before but that also there is something unknown beside it. I was shocked and very disappointed. She said that they would keep an eye on it with a scan within 2 months. It may be an infection or something else new. I shook hands with her and left the room feeling so low. I was glad that Gaz was with me. We chatted for a while. Gaz left and I went to make my next appointment in 4 weeks time. I then went to transport to go home. I had an hour to myself to think as I was upset. My mind was both blank and yet full of torment. I just knew that it would not be like before. My progress was flattened. My mind was a mess. I felt alone and that is when I knew that my fight was now suddenly bigger than ever. My fight was certainly not over. I said to myself "I told you so". I was annoyed and mad by all those people who mean well by saying "well done Dave"… "You'll beat it", and so on. "Listen to me … I cannot beat it, I can only delay its progress". I got home and it took me a few days to put it on Facebook. I was going to close the book here but there is so much to tell yet. It has been my endless journey from diagnosis, prognosis, treatment and where I am today. It has been an eventful journey and it's not over yet but I have to stop somewhere. I will however carry on for at least another couple of months. My story must be told and shared. I hope it helps people, families and friends. I am glad that I can share my cancer journey with you all, I enjoy putting it together. Please look for me on Facebook when my story ends in this book, but for now I am carrying on writing and tapping on my laptop. May your God look after you. Thank you … Dave xx.

——— # # # ———

Now this is the bit where we carry on and believe me, it is a rollercoaster of a ride. So here we go readers … on Friday JUNE 22nd 2018. I had my treatment today. Tonight my brother Liam arrived. He already knew from the Wednesday night of my latest situation and he has seen a terrible change in me. Yes, I have deteriorated an awful lot but that's what cancer and treatment does to you when it takes hold. As I said earlier in the book, the treatment is very often worse than the cancer itself. I have however decided to carry on fighting. Mr Bell in Kings College Hospital has ordered an MRI scan. I hate MRI scans as they are so claustrophobic, which for me is terrifying. I am convinced that in a previous life I was hanged and recovered to be then buried alive. Who knows. I hate having my neck being touched and I hate been enclosed in a closed area like a box or tight space.

——— # # # ———

SATURDAY JUNE 23rd. My brother Liam stayed last night and we had a chat like no others. Basically I laid out to him my life, my thoughts, my pains, my worries, my fears and hopes for the future. Whenever I do pass away, my family will be first on the mark. We chatted till 2.30am and by the time he left this afternoon we both knew so much about each other for the first time in years.

——— # # # ———

MONDAY JUNE 25th 2018. I was to attend the Lympadema clinic today but they cancelled. As far as I am concerned, during my entire treatment, they have been the most unhelpful bunch of scroats that I ever met. It's all about ticking the boxes just for the sake of it. Every time I go there one of them gets me on a seat and they begin to stroke my facial cheeks. They might as well stroke my ass cheeks. After fifteen minutes she always says "look at that, it looks better already". Rubbing my ass cheeks would have come up with a better result. That's it for the Lymphadema Clinic but they will need to see me in a few weeks from now or months if I can help it. As I said they are the only ones who want to simply tick the boxes. It annoys me when they constantly cancel appointments and without checking my treatment days, they then make new appointments which I always have to change as they just do not fit in with my other arrangements.

——— # # # ———

On THURSDAY JUNE 28th 2018. I attended Kings College Hospital and saw Mr Bell at 2pm. He told me that he can do no more for my back etc but referred me to another neurologist.

——— # # # ———

JULY 2018 was a busy month. I began to seriously look for someone to proof read my book. On July 2nd I met Jo in St Christopher's Hospice previously Harris Hospice near Orpington Hospital. Again I see no success here.

——— # # # ———

TUESDAY JULY 3rd 2018. My neck and back are giving me so many problems now. I curse the day when I broke it last year. Taking Morphine at 130mls every 12 hours with a top up of liquid morphine makes my day bearable now. My head is now tilted forward which puts pressure on my back and makes the pain sometimes unbearable. Friday July 6th 2018 is treatment day number thirteen(13). My treatment as you know is NIVOLUMAB Immunotherapy and is every two weeks on Fridays in The New Cancer Centre. It's a stunning place and so relaxing. Downstairs in the Transport lounge is so easy going and relaxing. Michelle and Fola are just so good here and put everyone at ease. I am so, so grateful for the transport there and back when I need it. Tuesday 10th … I went to my GP and met a Dr L at 9am. At 10am I had a physio appointment about my neck and back. My RIG site and feed tube is giving problems again so on 12th I had it replaced in the PRUH in Intervention Radiology. Thank you Stacey and Lynne. I was in at 8.45am and it was all over at 9.45am. My good neighbour Ian dropped me off and also picked me up. They live opposite and are so good to me. They cannot do enough for me. What wonderful neighbours to have. I am so lucky to have them nearby. Monday July 30th. I had a CT Scan in St Thomas'Hospital at 12.15pm and tomorrow at St Christopher's in Orpington I have another appointment. Keeping busy is part of the game.

——— # # # ———

AUGUST 2018 … A new month so let's see how many problems we have this month. On today Wednesday August 1st 2018, consultant and blood test not needed, The blood test itself is done on Friday morning but I have to get in early and as soon as results are back and satisfactory, then and only then will treatment begin in full. This Palliative care is not bad. I go to The New Cancer Centre once every two weeks for treatment. It's a small price to pay to be able to stay alive because of the treatment.

On Thursday 2nd I had an appointment with my GP Practice nurse in her treatment room at the actual practice. She called out my name with a lovely smile that she has naturally anyway but unknown to me, she had a hidden agenda lined up for me. I went into her room behind her and took a seat. I went to see her to look at and change the dressing on the site of my RIG tub, which is still in place. It was also a possibility that she might call my GP into the treatment room when the time came to change the dressings. She had a lovely surprise for me at first which had to be done in the form of two needles containing small amounts of a clear liquid. I suspected that one might be a big ass kicking flu jab in the shape of a sharp scratch. The other one was totally unexpected in that it was a Pneumonia jab. One was bad enough, but two needles in the space of a few minutes for me a person that detests needles was a nightmare but which had to be done. We decided to get both done and out of the way. It was done as swiftly as it was planned. I then thought will it protect me from flu and pneumonia, I have no idea but like my cancer treatments, I believe the medical experts. I then asked her to look at my RIG and the dressing that covered it and change it. She removed the dressing. It was a mess and leaking everywhere. I can't imagine what it's going to be like when the tube is going to come out. This will happen very soon as I eat and drink normally now so I am actually looking forward to having it removed. I was also very sore and the leaking was burning my abdomen. Inside it is amazing what the stomach actually puts up with as the gastric fluids break down the food and does not damage the stomach lining but as soon as a hole is created which was what happened to me when the feed tube was inserted, there was always the danger that when the time came to close that hole, it might not heal and not actually close itself. This was now getting out of hand and as the tube is still in place the hole is leaking enough to cause a burning pain. The practice nurse did all she could and dressed the area of the wound. It did not, however, solve the problem and I left the doctor's surgery with a new dressing and the contents of two injections in my upper left arm.

——— # # # ———

On AUGUST 7th 2018. I had a 10.30am appointment with Cardiology in the PRUH. It went well and they changed my heart medication. They also gave me a follow up appointment for Thursday August 16th 2018. In the meantime over the next week or so the arm that had been injected with two needles began feeling very sore and heavy, like a weight was put into it. My RIG site is giving major problems. I am now changing dressings four or five times in every twenty four hours. The gastric contents continue to pour out and burn my abdomen. Bleeding is then a major consequence if the dressings are not changed in time. It is amazing what the stomach puts up with from all this gastric acidic contents that only burn the abdomen and not in the stomach. It does burn the track on the way out but it has to stop soon. My abdomen is bleeding and is a mess. I want the tube out and the hole to be sealed up for good. Take for example what happened this afternoon. You all know me by now that I do not hold back about what I have gone through. There is no point in me tapping out on my laptop about my experience. I have of course not named people to protect those who requested not to be named. There are of course many people who are wonderful and have given me permission to use their full names. I must not divert away from what happened to me and my incident of gastric contents leaking and its consequences. Anyhow I was in the garden this afternoon in my garden swing seat laying down and just thinking of nothing and yet everything. I must have nodded off which was easy to do when the warm breeze of the afternoon was now and again interrupted by a light wisp of hot air that was trying to take over from the breeze, but the breeze came back and my balmy afternoon continued. I cannot remember but I may not at one stage be fully asleep but it was peaceful enough to let me hear the bees in the bush behind me, looking and sharing the nectar in the planted Dahlias and wild roses nearby. I could sometimes hear the birds nearby at the bird feeder and in the bushes behind me as they queued up to swoop across the garden and feed. Then it all ended as I fell asleep again, a process repeated several times during the blissful, warm balmy afternoon. It was an afternoon that I didn't want to end and yet I knew that when it did end, it would be repeated again the next day and the next day and so on. I have no idea how long I had been asleep but I woke up to find on the front of my shirt was a huge mass of Bluebottle Flies feeding on my stomach contents leaking from the dressing over the site of my abdomen. All around I noticed a mass of flying Bluebottles and other flies waiting their turn to feed on my leaking dressing. Then I realised that lately I was seeing more flies around me and now I knew why. I knew there and then that the site had to be closed up soon. How awfully embarrassing it would have been if it had happened at the same time if I was with family and friends. So this explains what happens when a person dies and is not found for a long time as the flies take over feasting on a corpse. Bloody hell, these flies are after me and I'm still alive. Go away flies, find someone else, I'm going nowhere. On the 9th I had a gastric band check up in the PRUH. All is well. On 10th I had a meeting with Yvonne my dietician in St Christopher's in Orpington. All is well and Yvonne is happy with my progress and also agrees with me that the RIG Tube should come out. That is the best news that I ever heard, as the next move should be to have the tube removed permanently. On Wed 15th I had an appointment with my Consultant in Guys and also had a blood test. My consultant is happy with my progress and suggested that I have a CT Scan soon.

On Thursday 16th I had my Cardiology appointment and he said he would consult my GP to change or increase my heart medication. Next Cardiology appointment will be on Thursday October 16th 2018.

On Friday 17th AUGUST 2018, I had my treatment of NIVOLUMAB Immunotherapy. There was nothing out of the ordinary and treatment went ahead at 8.30am. I have a procedure here now and as soon as my name is called,

I go in with a tea that I have been given as soon as I check into the Department for my treatment. After checking in, they tell me which Suite (A, B, C or D) that my treatment will be in. They take my appointment card and during treatment they enter the future appointments that I have here in The New Cancer Centre. Meanwhile, as I said, they call my name and I go into whatever suite is allocated to me. I chose any recliner and plug in my phone charger. The tea is put on the table and I sit down, headphones out and plugged in and then it's up to the cancer nurses to do the blood pressure etc. After a cannula is fitted, then a line of flush goes in over 20 minutes. When this is over and depending on Pharmacy, my infusion of NIVOLUMAB starts and goes in over the next hour or so while I listen to whatever, with my feet up. Sometimes the flush does not start if Pharmacy, for one reason or another, have not prepared my treatment. Anyhow treatment starts and after an hour or so the after flush starts. After a couple of hours it's all over and I leave the Department with extra fluid and a bag full of Immunotherapy Chemicals that I hope will make a big difference as it builds up within me and gives me extra time on this planet. I'm not ready to go yet but, it's not down to me to decide when that moment will be.

——— # # # ———

TUESDAY AUGUST 21st 2018. Finally the wait is over as R my Nutricia nurse is here in my home to remove the RIG tube from my abdomen. It was all over in a few minutes. She dressed the wound and left. It feels so weird now but am so glad that it's finally been removed. Now I need it to heal over but that is a lot to ask. It should start healing over in 4 to 6 hours but somehow I think that in my case it will take longer, much longer. Tuesday August 21st 2018 and today I feel a little stronger than normal so I ventured into sunny Bromley. I have a wedding to go to on Saturday September 1st 2018, so I think it's time anyway to splash out on a new suit etc. I went into the same place that I bought my previous suit from. I knew what I wanted so after fitting etc, I paid for it and left. They recommended a shop nearby that does alterations. I shuffled there as my feet and back were now hurting but my walking stick was a great help in the circumstances. After the measurements were taken I returned to my car. On the way there I went into M&S and bought some shoes etc. It was getting late but I enjoyed my day shopping which I hadn't done for a long time. I got home to a well earned mug of tea and of course some Morphine for pain relief. I have to be so careful with Morphine and not take any when, or before driving.

——— # # # ———

WEDNESDAY AUGUST 22nd 2018. This morning I have major problems in my abdomen as no healing happened overnight and gastric fluid and contents

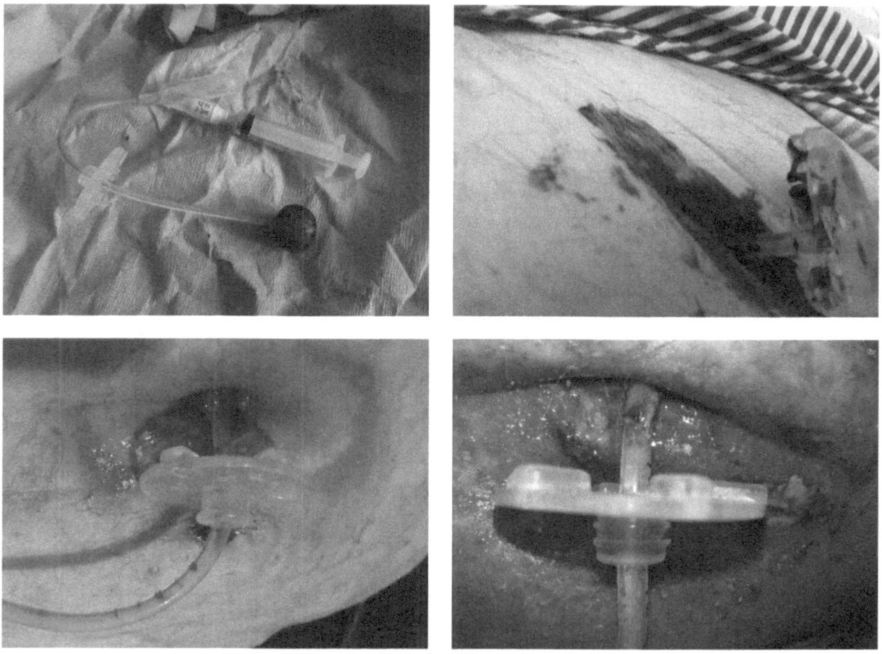

Problems with my RIG tube.

poured out of the hole and burned my abdomen. Overnight I changed dressings three times and will have to do it again in an hour or so. The pain is awful as it burned my skin. On 27th I called R my nurse and there was nothing she could do which I appreciate as in some cases it does take a long time, sometimes weeks. I can't go on for weeks like this not knowing when it will heal completely. On 28th I went to my appointment in St Christopher's in Orpington who advised me the same. Now the site of the wound is bleeding as my skin burns. I now know that I have an infection inside in the track. After that appointment, I took some clothes and a couple of old suits belonging to Garreth to the Cancer charity shop in Orpington. The suits were good quality so they were pleased with them. I was fully aware of my Rig site bleeding and leaking onto the dressings which are meant to protect my skin and clothes from burning and damage. It was a busy morning as I returned to Bromley to pick up my altered new suit. It fitted perfectly and I left there with a little smile on my face, something which has been missing for a while. Now I have Dina and Andrew's wedding coming up in the Barbican Centre in Central London on September 1st. I can't remember the last wedding that I went to, so this will be nice. Gaz is coming with me on the day. I got home and soon needed Morphine but all was now okay as regards pain control for the next few hours. I take morphine as my pain relief for my back but it has no effect on the burning of my abdomen. This cannot continue. There was no blood test or consultant on Wednesday 29th but on Friday 31st in Guys I had a blood test at 8.30am followed by treatment at 11am when blood test results took so long to come back. Okay … here we are now in September and the site is still leaking badly and burning me. Today, however, is Saturday September 1st 2018 and I have to do something soon. It is wedding day for my friend Dina and her future husband, Andrew. I awoke early in the morning as the plan is that I meet Garreth and we both then drive to the wedding venue. I had planned to leave home by 10am to pick up Gaz between 11 and 11.30am and then drive to The Barbican and the wedding. I heard the alarm on my phone go off and the back pain required me to take a small dose of Morphine. I dragged myself out of bed and after switching off alarm and unlocking locked doors, I quickly showered. I was fully aware of time slipping by but I was on schedule. I had already ironed a shirt last night and all was well until I suddenly let out a small howl of shock, horror and utter dismay on realising that my brand new suit was not where it should be in the wardrobe. It was just as well that the curtains were closed because picture the scene, a 61 year old male in a white shirt, black socks and blue pants running around the house looking for my new light blue suit. I have to find this suit, otherwise no wedding is happening for me. That was the whole reason that I bought the suit. I found the shoes but that was it. I was panicking. It was stupid panicking as I looked in places that no sane person would look for a suit. I was hobbling around like a headless chicken. I even looked under beds and then it hit me, charity shop, mix up in suit. Is my new suit in the charity shop all this time since the 28th of last month. Did they put it out with the other suits and if so it could be sold by now. Can you imagine, someone lucky may have just got a £100 suit for £12 or so. I rang the shop about my predicament and they confirmed that the suits that I gave them were out on the rack and one of them had been sold already. She then said that she would take the other suits off the rack and that I could come in and reclaim my new suit. I hung up after I thanked her. I broke out in a cold sweat and then out of the corner of my right eye I noticed a dry cleaning plastic cover from the dry cleaners that did the alterations. I looked in it and my life recovered when there it was all along, my new suit in a bag different to a normal suit protector bag. I was so, so relieved but I aged years with the shock of what could have been. I called the lady back to tell her the good news and that she could put the suits back on the rack to be sold. My day had been saved and soon I was in my new suit and off to the wedding.

——— # # # ———

THURSDAY SEPTEMBER 6th 2018. I went to my GP after getting an emergency appointment. He gave me a referral letter and I went home, packed a bag and went to A and E about 2pm. I was seen within 30 minutes and by 6pm I was in a cubicle but being attended to. I was back in hospital again. I spend a lot of time here but as time goes by things are going wrong more and more. Anyhow, I eventually got a bed in a medical ward which was a gastro ward under Dr A. I was told that he was the best at his work. The next morning after I had a very uncomfortable night with other patients in pain just like I was in pain. I take morphine at home but, so far, no doctor has written me up for morphine. In the meantime it's Paracetamol and a little injection to kill the pain but even together have no effect whatsoever on my pain which is now coming from an open hole in my stomach and from which leaks my gastric fluid and gastric contents and from my back which I broke late last year. My medical file is bloody huge and getting bigger every day. I have two huge files, one for The PRUH here and one for my Cancer in Guys and the nearby New Cancer Centre. As I said before, I therefore have also two different hospital numbers. The annoying thing is that the two different trusts argue and have in the past argued over sharing information which would otherwise have helped me and I would not have suffered needless pain and missed treatments. Anyhow now let us hope that things improve from now on. A temporary stoma bag was attached to the outside of my belly over the hole to collect all that pored out of the hole. Over the next few days, I was nil by mouth simply to rest my stomach. Gradually my nourishment was by drip only just to maintain my fluid levels and of course as a result the stoma bag was collecting less and less gastric contents. I was told by the team that the hole was healing itself and I would be discharged soon to recover in my home with those dreaded district nurses coming in to check on me and change dressings, if necessary. Ever since a district nurse demolished my letterbox and posted it back to me through the hole, then diving into a getaway car in a scene that Tom Cruise would relish as a stunt before the remainder of my letterbox had reached ground level with a crash, District nurses and I do not get on. Let me put it this way, they are not on my Christmas card list and will never ever be on one. On the 11th of September there was no option but to cancel my physio for later that day. I also cancelled my appointment to see my consultant and blood test for Wednesday 12th. Later on in the day of the 11th after 5 days not only did they remove the stoma bag but they also said that I could eat and drink normally but that I could also go home. I felt that it was too soon and the wound was not properly healed. (R I P to Raymond who passed away in the corner bed of my ward. What a nice guy, but no more pain now). I felt that very soon my RIG Site would leak again soon and be as bad as ever.

——— # # # ———

FRIDAY SEPTEMBER 14th 2018. I kept my appointment to have NIVOLUMAB treatment at 11.30am. It was a rushed morning as at 8am I had a blood test. At 8.15am was Lymphadema Clinic and from which I was discharged. While I waited for my blood test results to come back, I went to the Chemotherapy Dept where I was to have my Immunotherapy infusion treatment. I was called in to take a recliner seat while waiting for my treatment came up from Pharmacy. Then from out of the blue came Theresa my lovely and great Consultant to have a chat and to see on my welfare after my 5 days in hospital in the PRUH. My legs are retaining a lot of fluid but I need to keep them raised more often. My treatment began at 12 noon and by the time I got home that late afternoon, I was wrecked.

——— # # # ———

SATURDAY SEPTEMBER 15th I was in extreme pain and by evening time I was in a mess. MY RIG site was leaking and burning my abdomen as bad as ever. By the Sunday it was hell and I was crying in agony as my skin burned all over my belly. I knew it would happen again soon and I am sure they knew it would happen soon again. On Monday 17th Nutricia collected the last of my liquid food as I no longer needed it. Gradually over the following week, things went from bad to worse as the leaking and burning got almost unbearable. It was bleeding and I was changing dressings 6 to 7 times every 24 hours. On the 18th, my work colleague Peter M passed away from cancer. On 26th my appointment with Consultant and blood test was cancelled at 4pm. My NIVOLUMAB treatment went ahead on the 28th as normal. I had suffered long enough now but my 61st Birthday was soon here on October 7th. Last year I spent my 60th birthday in hospital and I was determined to have this 61st Birthday at home. October 7th. Happy 61st Birthday to me. I did not eat since yesterday as any food would mix with gastric fluids and leak out within an hour. I did however manage to have some chocolate birthday cake and it was lovely. An hour later however, the cake and some gastric acidic contents came out the hole and into the dressing. You may ask about how I know if it came out, well I hold nothing back about. I had eaten nothing that day so nothing had come out into the dressing but after dark chocolate liquid mixed with dark gastric acidic fluid leaked out then I knew that it was my stomach contents. There was no point in eating as it only leaked out and burned my abdomen to the point where I was crying with the extreme burning pain and the bleeding mixed with leaking clear fluid. I was waking up at night up to now changing dressings every 2 hours or so. When a grown man cries out in pain, then it's time to act. I decided to wait until morning and it's a day after my birthday.

——— # # # ———

MONDAY OCTOBER 8th 2018.... Good morning all and I have an appointment with my GP at 10am. When he saw it, he was visibly shocked. This was a repeat of what happened before. I asked in the morning for a doctor's referral letter. He also phoned the surgeon on call in the hospital. They were therefore, as a result of the phone call, expecting me in the PRUH. I left my GP surgery with the all important referral letter. On the previous hospital referral, I was seen quickly so I can only hope to be seen again as quick, but also that this time they finally sort it out, once and for all.

On arriving home I made a few phone calls and one of my lovely neighbours A, a couple of doors away from me, told me that she could take me into A and E at about 2pm to 2.15pm. All my neighbours are so, so good and have always been there for me. I completed packing my bag and yes at 2.15pm A came to me, as I was now shuffling rather than walking because of severe pain and a leaking dressing that had only been put on twenty minutes earlier. It was purely gastric fluid leaking out and it happens as soon as I bend forward. I cannot help bending forward ever since I broke that back bone last year. I managed to get into her car and we got to A and E in a few minutes. A helped me out of the car and with my two bags I shuffled into A and E and up to the counter. The tears were welling up in my eyes and I just could not hold back those tears any more. I was glad in a way to be here, I ran out of time, options, ideas and my hand was forced by the fact that I had now stopped eating. My pain relief which is Morphine 130mgs every 12 hours in granules plus when needed 20mgs of liquid Morphine every 4 to 6 hours. I say when needed but I do need it every 4 hours. Now that the morphine and any liquid pain relief is pouring out the hole, there is no pain relief in my body. I explained as easy as possible and as quickly as possible my predicament and not having pain relief since yesterday the 7th. I tried to explain that if I sat down or bent forward, the gastric fluid, the skin burning fluid would leak or pour out and burn me further. She nodded and said that "you will be called soon". Then in the same breath, it was like she had not listened to a single f*****g word that I had just said. I realised then that I was just a statistic and it was a case of move on, next please. I say this because what I said had fallen on deaf ears as she said to me "Take a seat, someone will call you soon". I told her that I will stand as fluid is leaking out. I walked away hoping for help. The tears still came but to save being seen to be a weak 61 year old, I was now screaming in agony. The burning was non stop as every move I made seem to make things worse. My pain is hell and in all honesty I just wanted to die there and then. My abdomen is red raw and as I looked into a now loose dressing I now also noticed blood as tiny blood vessels in my abdomen cannot take the burning acid from my stomach any more and have no option but to bleed. I was called after 20 minutes and was taken into a small assessment room and had my blood pressure etc, checked. After answering all the important questions and telling the two nurses that I cannot sit because of leaking gastric burning liquid, still nobody offered to change the dressing on the wound. I again was told to take a seat but one of the nurses then said that she realised that I could not sit but I had to wait outside and I would be called as quick as possible. That was the moment when I noticed the difference between a caring nurse and a civilian staff member on the counter frontline of A and E. Five minutes later another nurse came and called me away from the waiting room. This A and E here today was rammed and I was later to find out how bad it was as I left the waiting room and shuffled with my bags through a door into a treatment area of small cubicles. The door closed behind me and what I didn't know was it would stay closed for me. I was not going to see the outside world again for a little short of two weeks and I suppose I knew that because I could not go on like this current situation and I was determined to stay until it was sorted. I was put into a cubicle and told to lie on a trolley. They told me they realised that the burning pain from stomach fluid pouring out was pretty bad as they had seen it before in a previous case. I got on the trolley and they put pillows under me while I eased myself onto the trolley and lay flat on my back. At first the fluid burned all around my abdomen and mixed with burst burnt small blood vessels, it was not a pretty sight. A lady appeared with blonde curly hair and a stethoscope around her neck and told me she was the Consultant/Surgeon on call, and she said she would be admitting me as the situation was too serious for me to go home.

She was there with a nurse and together they changed a dressing for a new one. My pain killers were well overdue but the usual excuse was applied in that as a doctor had not written them onto my file etc, I could not have them yet. The Consultant/Surgeon then looked through my medication in my bag and put them on my system. Things were looking up, or at least I thought they were. As I lay flat on my back, the burning pain eased as the damaging burning acid flowed backward and back into the hole in my abdomen and down back into the track and into my stomach. As long as I lay on the flat of my back, there was no leaking acid and therefore no pain. The fact that the pain had gone for now was like a new lease of life. The Consultant/Surgeon went away but not before telling me that she was now going to look for a bed for me anywhere in the hospital. It was a bad day to be in A and E and no beds were available anywhere in the hospital, so when she returned fifteen minutes later, that is exactly what she told me. She then told me that the cubicle that I was in was needed as it was part of the treatment area attached to A and E and as I was now past that part of the hospital treatment area, and someone would come and move me soon. She left but did however inform me that she would locate me later, wherever I ended up. Within a few minutes a hospital porter came to me with a yellow hospital wheelchair and told me that we were on the move.

The time was just before 3.15pm on Monday October 8th 2018. I had been here for just under an hour and now I was on the move. I asked him where we were going but as he loaded my bags onto the chair with my walking stick, he made no reply to my question. I asked him again and he said that we were going to a waiting area. As I eased myself off the trolley onto the chair, the burning acid began leaking out and doing its damage to be again. I screamed in agony and held my dressing away from the skin of the burnt area. I was taken to a room, yes a room with four walls, a door and a sink. On a wall was a bracket where a TV had once upon a time had a place of pride to keep patients and visitors entertained. As I looked around me, there was a small collection of five other patients in hospital chairs. I say patients, but we were actually a collection of human debris wrapped in blankets. I had no idea what their reason was for being here. I asked a nurse as to how long we would be here and all she said was that she needed to get me a wristband. She walked away and came back ten minutes later with wristbands for me and a few others in the room.

Without me asking, she put on my wristband and then said that we would be here for quite a while as there were no other beds or cubicles available anywhere in the hospital. I didn't say it but no doubt, there was availability in the mortuary. She then put on the wristbands on a few other patients and I couldn't forget that as all of us "human debris" awaited beds for our various ailments, we were actually dependent on other forms of "human debris" elsewhere in the various wards being discharged home or some poor sod reaching the end of their life and actually being taken to the mortuary. I dare say the time will come one day as I, with my terminal cancer, may be in a ward somewhere dying and people like me or those around me will be depending on my death and transferred to the mortuary. I dread the thought of it but I cannot forget that it may be the case.

Anyhow, back in our little room, the time was now near 6pm. I had been bent forward, but no movement. I had sips of water as anything more would have triggered movement of burning gastric acid. Time dragged on and no sign of movement yet. No beds available and the noise all around was so loud, people swearing and shouting, I knew however that I had to stick it out and going home was not an option. At about 9pm there was movement as a lady opposite me in a chair was moved from the room by a porter. I can only assume that a bed had become available in a female only ward. I nodded of again. I soon found myself in very severe pain, a burning pain that was not easing off at all, In fact, if anything this pain was getting worse and still no pain relief because when I asked I was told that even though the doctor/consultant had written up my medications to the system in my name she had authorised, but not written up the morphine that I normally have to kill severe pain. All I had as pain relief written up for me was Paracetamol. That may be okay as a painkiller for a tooth ache but right now it is totally useless to ease the pain of gastric acid pouring out of my stomach through a hole that will not close and as a result is physically burning my belly and is damaging as well as destroying clothes such as shirts.

There was still no movement on the issue of being given a bed. At about 11.15pm, the nurse who was looking after us all in the room then began her rounds of observations such as temperature checks and blood pressure checks. There was now a small group of four of us in this room. Before this nurse came to do her observations, it was beginning to look like we had been forgotten about. Anyhow now that we "were found" as such, it was soon my turn to be checked. I had my hands across the front of my abdomen. The fluid was leaking out and even though I needed a new dressing on it, that would have to wait until after the observations had been completed. It was hell as I had to straighten up while the blood pressure cuff was put on my right arm. I screamed and then cried out in agony while I sat up in the chair. As the already saturated dressing touched my belly, new fluid poured out and burned my skin. There was nowhere to go, I just sat here and screamed as it got worse and worse. I needed Morphine but as yet nothing on the system for me. All observations done and I asked for my dressing to be changed. I soon bent forward again to find my comfortable position where nothing rubbed against my open stomach wound and its access track to outside my abdomen. I asked for a change of dressing and as I waited for the nurse to come back to do it and as I was leaning forward, the already over saturated wound dressing could take no more. Gastric fluid, gastric contents and a mixture of both blood and liquidised gauze came out. Also, mixed with that was and pouring out was a strange mix of foul smelling blood and liquidised flesh from the track out from stomach to the open world. There was now nothing in its way as it just dripped on to the floor. There was a call button near the sink in the corner and a visitor to one of the other patients pressed it. Things had now reached a peak. The nurse came in a few minutes later and with a dressing in her left hand, she just looked at the mess on the floor and told me she would get help. She returned five minutes later with another nurse who was responsible for bed managing. It was obvious now that my situation was a priority. The time was a little after midnight and soon I was told that I would be on the move. A new dressing was put on the open leaking wound and a cleaner was soon mopping up.

My tears were still flowing as I lifted my feet for the cleaner to mop around my feet. At about a quarter past midnight, a porter appeared and told me that I was on the way to Medical Ward Nine. Like a pack horse, my bags were loaded on to my yellow hospital chair and off we went. I had no idea where it was but it had to be better than this NHS approved holding area. The nurses, doctors all staff had so much to do and they done it with pride, dedication and an individual love and care for each and every patient, but they need so much more staff and an injection of Government investment. I got to the ward in a matter of minutes.

The time was now near 0.30am on Tuesday October 9th 2018. It had taken a little over 9 hours from walking up to the counter in A and E to getting into a bed in a proper ward, but I thought about what it took to get moved. I had to endure the pain both mental and physical as well as the embarrassment of strange types of gastric contents dripping on to the floor in front of other patients and their helpers and carers. I was so glad to be soon lying on a bed in a proper ward. Soon two nurses came to clean up the wound again. No dressing was put on it as instead a Stoma bag was fitted around the hole to collect anything that came out of the open track wound. I was helped out of my clothes and into a hospital gown. I laid flat on the bed and the pain eased. All contents was now coming out and into the stoma bag. That was the whole plan. It was a little like before with the same problem but this time they know it has to be sorted before I an discharged. I wanted to be in hospital to get it sorted so I expect that this will be the end result. I soon realised that also I was "nil by mouth". This was so that nothing goes in and therefore the stomach would be soon empty. An empty stomach means no contents coming out into the Stoma bag. It would take around four or five days nil by mouth to see results. In the meantime, I was connected up to a drip and my fluid intake was maintained throughout. My morphine was at last put on the system for me and I gladly accepted it when it was offered to me. The pain soon eased and I began to realise that I was going to get through all this. I was in good hands here with Nurse Maria from Greece looking after me.

On Wednesday 10th, I was moved to Medical 6 which was a proper Gastro Ward. The same wonderful care that I had in Medical 9 continued in Medical 6. One of my consultant's team Dr Philip checked on my progress every day. A plan was put together to add acid reducing medication to my list. Gradually the stoma bag was collecting nothing. I had an ultra sound test and had to swallow a camera to see what exactly was going on in there and to see if the hole in my stomach was actually closing up naturally. If not, it was planned to operate and while in there, the hole would be closed with whatever they close holes like what I have. Obviously my visit to see my consultant on Wednesday 10th and Immunotherapy treatment on Friday 12th was all cancelled until I am out of hospital and at home. I was also allowed to eat normally and drink normally on the 11th. I was so hungry so to eat was heaven. There was now nothing leaking out into the stoma bag and I could feel myself getting better. I was weighed also today on Friday 12th and I soon realised that the day I came into Medical 9, I was 70 kilos. Today I am 63.5 kilos. I was also visited by Maria from Medical 9 and, of course, we had a good chat about Greece and of course my heaven on earth, Skiathos. My worst experience has got to be what happened on Saturday October 13th while in Medical 6, I was told that I would have to have a GASTROGRAFIN test. Let me tell you that this test is a test that if in the wrong hands, can do a lot of harm or should I say it can do a lot of harm if in the wrong intestines etc. It all began at about 7pm on that Saturday evening. My nurse in charge at the time came to me during the handover to night staff, which was just before she finished her long crazy twelve hours plus shift. She told me that I was to have a GASTROGRAFIN test later on that night. I had no idea what she was talking about, or what was involved as she picked up a bottle from her medication trolley and gave it to me. She told me that I was to take it in a container mixed with water. In total I think it was about a half pint of liquid and I drank it there and then in front of the nurse that gave it to me. I was then told that in four hours time after drinking it all, porters would take me down to Radiology. The nurse then told me that the liquid lights up everywhere it goes to and therefore any leaks in the stomach, intestines or bowel would become obvious to see in the Radiology Department in an x ray. It had a strange smell similar to Emulsion paint and tar. Innocently, I drank the foul smelling liquid as quick as possible so as not to prolong the event any further than necessary. It certainly was foul smelling and foul tasting. However, there was going to be a bad sting in the tail, yes my bloody tail. As I had swallowed all the liquid at about 7.20pm, I was therefore expecting to be taken down to the Radiology Department at around 11.20pm. It was a weekend though and it would have been busy so I was expecting them to be coming for me later than expected. I just lay on my bed and waited for them to arrive. The sting in the tail is on the way. Barely two hours had passed when I suddenly felt a rumble in my stomach that was unexpected but not strange. After a further twenty minutes the rumbling got worse and I suddenly pictured that lovely nurse looking at her watch in the comfort of her home and smiling at my current experience that she probably knew about but had not told me. I however knew full well what was happening and as the rumbling got louder and louder, I thought to myself "My God, my life is ending", Nobody told me it was an enema. In all my sixty one years I have never known an enema to work this quick, but now I do. I took off like "a scalded cat" as my internal Satellite Navigation kicked in to direct me to the nearest toilet. I made it on time as I quickly shut and bolted that door behind me and adopted that position that I had no intention of vacating for a long, long time. It happened and it felt like all my internal organs shifted position inside me. It was so bad, I didn't know what part of my body my ass had moved to. I sat there for thirty minutes as my whole life drained down the toilet bowl. There was nothing left inside me, or so it felt that way. It was so bad, I was surprised that none of my internal bone structure had left me to disappear as well down the toilet bowl. Without being too graphic, but I suppose it is too late for that, it was liquid torture. I was lucky that in this toilet there was also a shower unit so I got myself cleaned up. I opened the door after getting dressed and returned to my bed. I got another towel ready just in case. Within seconds, the experience was to be repeated. I went straight for the same toilet/shower and again, after locking the door behind me, repeated the earlier procedure. It was not as bad and after another fifteen minutes or so the event reached another closure. I again got showered and cleaned up and left again to return to my bed. The first thing on my mind was to grab my phone and even though it was too late for a warning, I had to "google" the word GASTROGRAFIN. There it was, its full explanation of the purpose of its use followed by the words "can also be used as an enema". Ah well, now I know. I laid back in my bed and waited for these porters to arrive.

I fell asleep until a night nurse woke me up to take observations at about 2am and also to tell me that a porter was waiting to take me down to Radiology Department and The Gastrografin Test. My God it's the early hours of Sunday morning. The porter and a night nursing assistant took me down there and told me that the reason for the late test was simply down to the fact that A and E was rammed and only a handful of porters available. As soon as I got there, the porter left to go elsewhere. I was taken in and after exchanging a few details, I was scanned by this machine that looked at everything inside me that was now glowing brightly thanks to GASTROGRAFIN. This scan experience lasted only a few minutes but we had to wait for another fifteen or twenty minutes until the same original porter came to return me to my bed in Medical 6. Back in my bed, I soon drifted off to sleep after being given some Morphine for pain. Breakfast was at 8am and I was starving.

Weekends are boring in hospital. Monday morning October 15th I was facing a camera test so again I was nil by mouth. At 2pm I was taken down to Endescopy to swallow a camera and see what was going on in there. I was now in the very capable hands of the same surgeon who done my Gastric Band back in 2009. At bedside my also very capable Doctor Philip was now looking after me and told me that this camera test would probably tell them a lot as to how soon I would be going home from here. In the Endescopy Department, I asked to be sedated when I saw the size of the camera and its unit that would be put down my throat and into my stomach. I remember nothing about it all and woke up in recovery at 4.15pm. I was returned to the ward but sedation had not fully worn off. I felt like crap but woke up at about 9pm and asked for something to eat. I was given a sandwich and a cup of tea. I soon felt a little better and after some morphine for pain relief, I soon drifted off to sleep.

Tuesday October 16th 2018, Good morning all. On reflection about yesterday and the size of that camera, I am relieved that they got the correct end of my body when inserting it. Doctor P came to see me and told me that there were no abnormalities in the stomach after the camera test. He also said that hopefully, surgery can now be avoided. There was however another test to undergo and it involved more swallowing on tomorrow Wednesday the th. I am fully expecting my old enemy GASTROGRAFIN to make a return visit More nil by mouth again and on Wednesday sure enough it was another swallowing test. I was taken down to Radiology again and met my two lovely nurses there Stacey and Lynne. I was relieved to be told that Gastrografin was miles away, well not exactly miles away, but in the Hospital Pharmacy. As far as

I am concerned Gastrografin can stay in the Pharmacy. The internal geography of my body was temporarily altered by Gastrografin, but all is okay now. The test was easy, as I had to swallow a clear orange flavoured liquid that again lit up all inside. The doctor there that did the test told me that all was okay with no leaks. He also said that he would immediately tell them in my ward that I was okay to go home soon. I was taken back to the ward and waited for the official okay to go home. Thursday 18th I had an appointment in Cardiology but they came up to the ward to see me. My Friday 19th appointment in Guys for treatment was cancelled and Dr P told me later in the day that I could go home. The small delay was to make sure that all was definitely okay to discharge me. I was discharged later on the evening of Friday 19th October 2018. Good morning all it's Saturday 20th 2018 and it is great to be home. The RIG site is now completely healed, no leaks. My days of leaking wounds and leaking dressings are now fully over. No more gastric fluid burning my skin and destroying clothes.

On Wednesday 24th I saw my consultant in Guys at 2.30pm. As much as I wanted to see Theresa, I saw instead one of her new team. All is well so far and despite my weight loss which was originally 70 kilos but now 64 kilos. It will soon recover now that I'm at home. My Friday treatment of NIVOLUMAB Immunotherapy went ahead as planned after a blood test at 8.15am. It did not happen however until near 10.30am after the blood test results came back. This was treatment number 20. Because of the recent gap in treatments as I was in hospital, the tiredness hit me hard and it took a few extra days to fully recover from it. I now also have an abscess in my left upper gum. Doctor gave me a course of antibiotics for it. The month of October ended quite. No major problems and we slipped into November quietly.

Friday November 9th 2018 was a mad, crazy, busy day. I was collected by transport just after 5.30am and got to Guys at 6.40am. Nothing was open until 8am so I put my head down and set the alarm on my mobile for 7.50am. I had my blood test at 8.05am which was followed by a CT Scan on my cancer at 8.45am. I then had my treatment at 9.30am. That was when they told me that there had been no need to have a blood test. I went to Transport after and was home by 12.50 in the afternoon.

On Wednesday 14th November 2018 at 11am, I attended the Zoledronic Acid infusion Department. I had an infusion of Zoledronic Acid to strengthen my bones. I had a similar infusion done this time last year after I had broken my back. As I left, one of the nurses that treated me said "Cheerio Mr Cosgrave, see you this time next year". I really do hope she is right, as I'd love to be alive obviously. I feel good at the moment apart from my back and neck problems. On Friday 16th I had a phone call assessment at 11am from my Physio just to keep them up to date. It was a great, helpful phone call and I explained to him that I had a Neurologist appointment in the PRUH at 2.30pm on Tuesday 20th

November. Another result of the meeting was a series of neck exercises.

Saturday 17th November, 18th and 19th all was well still. I am anxious about my Neurologist appointment today November 20th. So far I have not really had much reaction from Consultants etc about my neck. Maybe Dr St***** would be different. I got there early and after giving in my appointment letter, I had just taken a seat and my name was called to have blood pressure etc, taken. When that was done, a female doctor came to me as I was returning to my seat and asked me to follow her to her Consultation room. She asked me to tell her what happened as regards my problem going back to last year etc. When I told her everything, she did a series of tests which lasted about 15 minutes. She was great and very thorough and I was both amazed and delighted when she said "Mr Cosgrave, I think we can help you with this". She then went on to explain that She would refer me to another specialist in Kings College Hospital who would administer injections to my neck muscles. To strengthen them. Then she surprised me when she told me the contents of those injections. Honestly, I could not believe it when she said I would be getting Botox injections which would be repeated every three months to be effective enough. Bloody Hell, I thought what next? I am now looking forward to my Botox sessions. It makes me feel like I am up there amongst how the rich and famous live, so bring it on as I'm really looking forward to it. I left there with a spring in my step as finally something positive seems to be happening. That spring in my step soon stopped when I found my car had been vandalised by someone running something very sharp along the driver side from back to front and then smashing my wing mirror on same side. No cctv and no witnesses, very annoying but I cannot let it get to me.

——— # # # ———

On WEDNESDAY NOVEMBER 21st 2018, I had a very important meeting with my Consultant. Normally I meet one of the team, but today was going to be my lucky day as I just spotted Theresa, my Consultant. My transport had arrived late and after I got some tea, I waited to be seen and get my scan results. I spotted Theresa again in the corner of my eye. My height and weight had already been taken so I soon saw my name to go to Room Number 1. It was nearby so I waited outside as I had seen Theresa just leaving that room a few minutes earlier. Theresa came back with a CNS and we all entered the room. Theresa looked at me and I got that smile from her, a reassuring smile. She then told me what I wanted to hear. She said that all was well, all was stable and the tumours etc were all stable. Thank God for NIVOLUMAB Immunotherapy treatment. It's working for me as it has been doing for the past few months with mostly all good scan results. I've been on this NIVOLUMAB Immunotherapy now for a year or so and as I said before, it's great that Theresa gave it to me all that time ago. She said that treatment and blood tests would continue and a CT Scan would be in February 2019. I left there and went downstairs to have a blood test as requested by Theresa. I was also now thinking that this Christmas 2018 would be a good one or at least better than last Christmas. This New Year 2018 into 2019 would also be special. A year is a long, long way away and who knows what will happen during the coming year. I am now used to the fact that things can go wrong even overnight. I was tired after today and transport was late as well. I didn't get home 'till 10pm and soon went to bed. On Friday I had my treatment as normal but again had transport that got me home late again at 7pm. I was wiped out also on Saturday morning after the treatment but was recovered by the late afternoon.

——— # # # ———

SUNDAY NOVEMBER 25th 2018, I feel good apart from my neck and back problems. I hate to admit to this but as Part 1 of this book was being proof read, that is now completed so this book will be closing soon in the coming days. On the 26th, I had some work done by putting in a new, upgraded bathroom, toilet etc. It was done over two days and looks great now. I arranged it because I feel upbeat about life at the moment and because I realise that without much warning it will end and then my life will be ending. On the 27th, 28th, 29th and 30th I began planning the ending of this book.

——— # # # ———

On FRIDAY NOVEMBER 30th I attended Guys to have a blood test at 8am and my NIVOLUMAB immunotherapy infusion treatment a couple of hours later after my blood test results came back. Very soon, leading up to Christmas, I am doing a number of activities to keep busy and active. Next week is my planning of a night out at the Christmas Panto which is coming up. This is followed by the return from the repair shop of my recently vandalised car. I am then with family and friends, going to the Tower of London for the Ceremony of the Keys. Following this is again family and friends going to Westminster Abbey and then Christmas with family and friends. I will enjoy every moment this Christmas because who knows what is around the corner. In my case, the Grim Reaper is never far away before I get that tap on the shoulder to say, "Thanks Dave, it is all over and your work here is done". Writing this book has taken over my life for the past couple of years and I am absolutely delighted to have done it. It was something that I felt needed to be done to tell everyone all that I went through. I hope it helps people. It has helped me to get all that was in my head into a book of what I am going through. If it happened, it's in here, nothing held back as I said, apart from some names of some people. The end of all of this experience is coming to an end for the purpose of this book.

As luck would have it, I assumed the book had come to an end, but, of course, I am delayed by the taxman while I register for a Unique Tax Reference number. In the meantime, the following happened. On December 3rd I had new fittings put in for a shower, toilet and bathroom. Wednesday December 5th and I had a Cardiology appointment, where all went well. New tablets to keep me alive. On Friday 7th I had my Immunotherapy appointment and all went very well. December 14th and I had an appointment with Yvonne, my Dietician, who is amazed with my progress. She also told me that there will be one more appointment on January 25th when she will discharge me. I am astonished myself. because it was only a few months ago that I thought I had my feeding tube fitted for life. Thanks to Theresa, I have transformed myself and now look forward to every day. I am still terrified by death but lets see eh! On Dec 20th myself, my Gaz with Natalie and her parents, together with family from abroad, went to the Ceremony of the Keys at the Tower of London. A great experience which was followed by Natalie's parents and her family inviting me to attend Westminster Abbey, on Christmas Eve, for the Christmas Service of carols and hymns etc. What an experience it was for me to dress up in my suit with a black overcoat and go inside the lovely Westminster Abbey on a very special night. I loved it all and felt wanted and alive. I spent Christmas with this lovely family of Gaz's girlfriend, Natalie. I enjoyed every minute as I do not know if I will be here for next Christmas. Please God I will, but no promises. I came home for New Year and on January 2nd, 2019, I went to Ireland for a couple of days. Ryanair from Standsted to Cork. My sister picked me up and after meeting Gaz and Natalie from the train station in Cork, we travelled over to west Cork. I stayed at the Clonakilty Park hotel and on the Thursday 3rd, my sister Mary took us all to Dingle, in Co Kerry. I saw the amazing 2km long Inch Beach and the Blasket Islands with Skellig Michael on the horizon, where part of *Star Wars* was filmed. Back in West Cork, I visited family members where I stood and said a prayer at my parents graveside. I went into the Church of The Assumption at Ahiohill and we lit candles. The weather was terrible on the 2nd but was dry by the time I had left there. We all returned back to UK on January 4th and my delayed Immunotherapy was given to me on the 8th January. There you go, we are up-to-date regarding my book. My luck is in – I have just had a letter for the taxman so I can now stop my diary.

I currently feel okay, not great, but every day that I wake up to is a good day. I look forward to waking up every morning whereas so many people do not want to wake up. Many people cannot and do not sleep. I also realise that, as time progresses, the reality of the cancer winning is looming. I am now about to begin my 6th year fighting off my death. Therefore, it has to happen soon. My only hope is research or another new life-prolonging drug to be offered to me. My current drug NIVOLUMAB will not be given to me after the end of

2019 so you can imagine how I depend on something that will work then. In the past, there were many moments that I wanted to die in my sleep, the painless way. It may be said that it could be described as the cowards way out but nobody dies in pain if it can be avoided. My condition, at the moment, is kept together with an awful lot of morphine which I take orally. The taste is disgusting but it controls the pain. My routine is a shot at 9am, again at 1pm, same repeated at 6pm and finally before bedtime at 11pm. I take nothing at night unless I wake with pain. I realise that I will lose the morphine when my neck and back problems are sorted but then the cancer may necessitate the return of that same Morphine. I have no pain from my cancer at the moment. I am therefore waiting for that day. I also realise now that as the time goes by, my cancer will more than likely cease being stable. It has been absolute hell from being diagnosed, through to the treatment in its various different stages. To quickly summarise, I would be dead by now if I hadn't met Theresa, my Consultant. She changed my treatment a few times to get the best that was available at the time. I was lucky that this wonderful lady Theresa Guerrero-Urbano had been put on this planet to help people. In my eyes, she is a walking saint who has devoted her life to do for people what she has done for me. I was given 18 months to live and even though as I said, that time was up on June 25th 2015, I simply ask one question, why am I still here? To this day, I still lie in bed at night thinking, crying and sometimes asking myself "why me" in the first place and now torturing my mind by keeping me on the edge between life and death. Recently I did something that I also did last year; I drove to Beckenham Crematorium, a few miles away from my home. I went in there and parked in the car park near the chapel. This is where it will end for me, whenever my luck runs out, I spent twenty minutes there, again thinking. I left there and took an easy journey home. It is something that I had to do and if my life is prolonged further after the next few scan results, I will do it again. In the pre-prepared envelope of my funeral wishes, this is the place that I want my funeral to be in. The funeral of my wife was held here so I too wish to be cremated in the same place. There are some photos in this book which are important to me. The cover is from my piece of heaven, Skiathos Island in Greece. There are also photos of me at some stages of my treatment when I was at my worst and I do hope never to go back to that ever again. Thank you all and please find me on Facebook. My profile photo is of Skiathos. I say this because if my condition deteriorates, I may not get a chance to pre-advise you all of my ending. I will never ever forget two events in my life as regards a close death in my family. I have already mentioned that when my lovely dad passed away, I missed his funeral simply down to me missing my flight because of heavy traffic. I did however get home to Ireland on time to be at my mum's bedside before she died. I cradled her head on one of my arms and whispered into her ear that she could go now to be with my dad, which is what she did shortly afterwards. Finally, my mum and dad were together again. It was there and then that I realised what a lovely way to leave this life and go to whatever is in the next life. I also experienced the same when my lovely wife Joan, at 46 years old, passed away peacefully back in 2008. I am absolutely terrified now of dying. It scares the life out of me and that feeling was different a few months ago. It is now early January 2019 but back in July or so, I was okay about dying. I was ready for bad results which never happened. I then became aware of the fact that maybe death was not going to happen when I expected it to happen. My mind was in turmoil because I then had to prepare to stay alive with death being put on the back burner so to speak. Now, as I get used to this experience of good stable results, I am now terrified of suddenly getting a result that could mean death in a matter of months. What then if that happens? It hurts my head to think about it. I do not want it to happen, but if in pain, it is a wonderful release. Now I realise that there is hell also for those I will leave behind, a hell on earth to what I believe, is a peaceful alternative. Cheerio my readers. Bless you all and keep the fight. This is it, until we meet again, GOODBYE! … Dave … xxxxx.

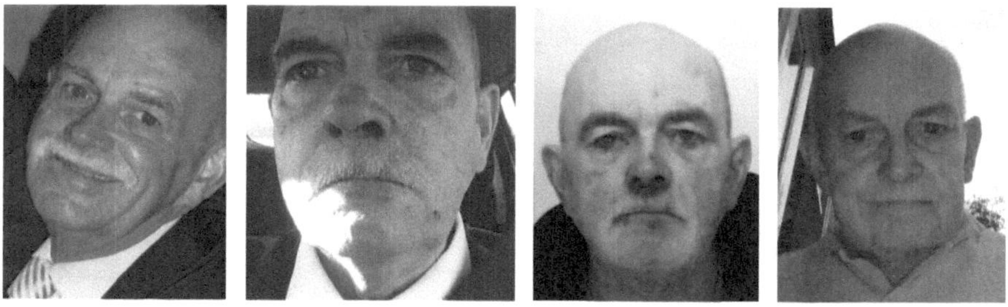

Then, and now.

Made in United States
Troutdale, OR
11/03/2026

56844694R00126